BEST HIKES AND WALKS OF SOUTHWESTERN BRITISH COLUMBIA

Revised and Updated

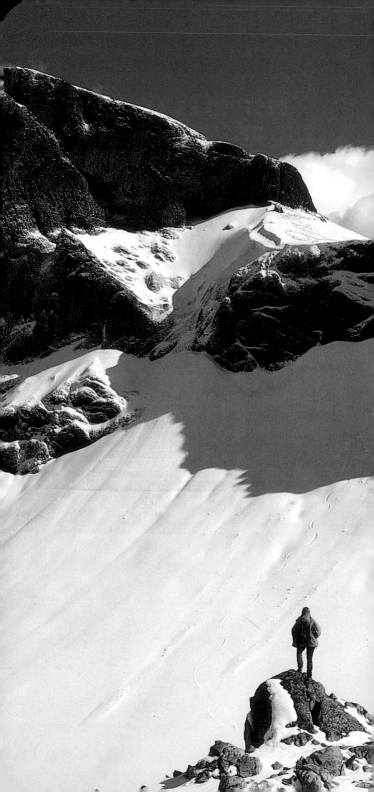

BEST
HIKES
and
WALKS
of
Southwestern
British Columbia

Revised and Updated

Dawn Hanna

LONE
PINE

The Publisher: Lone Pine Publishing

10145 – 81 Avenue	1808 B Street NW, Suite 140
Edmonton, Alberta	Auburn, Washington
Canada T6E 1W9	USA 98001

Senior Editor: Nancy Foulds
Editor: Jill Fallis
Production Manager: David Dodge
Cartography: Volker Bodegom
Design, Layout and Production: Carol S. Dragich, Gregory Brown
Separations: Elite Lithographers Co. Ltd., Edmonton, Alberta, Canada

All photos by the author except the following:
Mark Haddock, 281
Greg Maurer, front and back covers, title, contents page (2 photos) 8, 18, 19, 104, 131, 169, 187, 188, 217, 236, 238, 240, 244, 245, 271, 272, 301, 302, 309, 310, 313, 319, 320, 325, 331, 342, 359
Michael Steig, 128
Greg Stoltmann, 164
Mia Stainsby, 192
Gavin Wilson, 191

Illustrations:
Birds & Animals: Gary Ross, 23, 29, 34, 41, 44, 57, 83, 89, 121, 170, 231, 249, 332
Tracks: Ian Sheldon, 21, 332

The publisher gratefully acknowledges the support of Alberta Community Development and the Department of Canadian Heritage.

PC: P13

DISCLAIMER

The hikes in this book are based in part on a series of columns originally published in *The Vancouver Sun*. Neither the *Sun* nor Pacific Press Ltd. nor Southam Inc. bear any liability for the information contained within.

Hiking, as with all outdoor activities, involves an element of the unknown and thus, an element of risk. Weather, erosion and other forces may change the conditions or route of a trail. Thus, keep in mind that this book serves as a guide only. It is the ultimate and sole responsibility of the reader to determine which hikes are appropriate to his or her skills or fitness levels or those of his or her party. Readers/hikers also hold the ultimate and sole responsibility to be aware and alert of changes and/or hazards that might have occurred since the research and writing of this book.

ACKNOWLEDGEMENTS

This book could not have been written without the assistance of many people, and to them I would like to give thanks. In no particular order, those people are:

Jim Cuthbert and Chris Tunnoch of BC Parks' Vancouver District Office; Drew Carmichael and Vicki Haberl of BC Parks' Garibaldi–Sunshine Coast District; Beth Wilhelm in the Victoria office of the Ministry of Environment, Lands and Parks; Mary Trainer and Sue-Ellen Fast of the Greater Vancouver Regional District Parks Department; Eric Lees of the West Vancouver Parks Department; Volker Bodegom of Lone Pine Publishing's Vancouver office for his meticulous attention to the maps contained herein; and Shane Kennedy and senior editor Nancy Foulds for making me feel like a part of the Lone Pine family.

A special thanks to Halvor Lunden for just being Halvor, which means being an inspiration in his energy and enthusiasm, and for his untiring work building and maintaining many of the trails in this book. To my mum Joanne Van Antwerp, dad Don Hanna and brother Scott Hanna, all of whom have abetted me on the trail. All my hiking buddies during the past few years, who are too numerous to mention, but especially my mountain mentor Larry Emrick.

And an extra special thanks for all the kilometres logged, weather endured, photographs taken and support given by my other mountain mentor, Greg Maurer.

CONTENTS

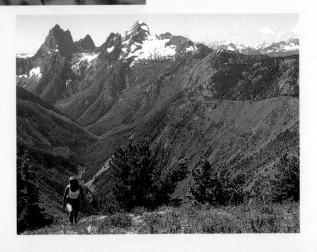

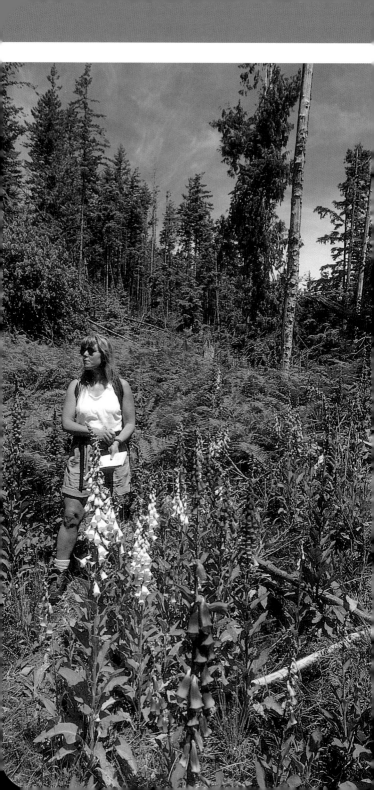

PREFACE

Early in 1996, I spent a month hiking the wild places of Patagonia, almost 15,000 kilometres from home. I was entranced by weird spires of pink granite, tiny Darwin's ostriches and impossibly blue glaciers that regularly heaved house-sized icebergs from their leading edge.

My constant companion was a tattered collection of the works of Henry David Thoreau. At first, it seemed strange to be reading of a rapture for the tame ponds and forests of New England in a place so wildly different. But later, Thoreau's ideas of the transcendent spirit of nature and of his passion for wild places helped me feel at home in a strange land.

At the same time, his words made me yearn for the beauty of British Columbia and its wild places—my wild places, the ones in which I had hiked for many years. And I discovered that although I could appreciate the beauty of distant peaks, aged beech forests and exotic wildlife, it could never match the wilderness in my own backyard. Nor could it touch me in quite the same way.

This book is part of an effort to bring to others what I have found in exploring the mountains, rivers, forests and fields of this province; and, I hope, to follow in the footsteps of Thoreau and live deliberately and learn what the woods have to teach.

In his 1862 essay 'Walking,' Thoreau writes: 'The West of which I speak is but another name for the Wild; and what I have been preparing to say is, that in Wildness is the preservation of the World.'

More than 130 years later, the words ring especially true. Throughout BC, a process is underway to decide which wild places will be preserved as parks and ecological reserves and which will be logged, mined or otherwise developed. The government has set 12 percent of BC's land base as the amount to be protected.

Public opinion has a tremendous impact on which areas will be set aside. Don't be shy about expressing passion for your wild places.

Dawn Hanna

Dawn Hanna and foxgloves, Mount Artaban Trail.

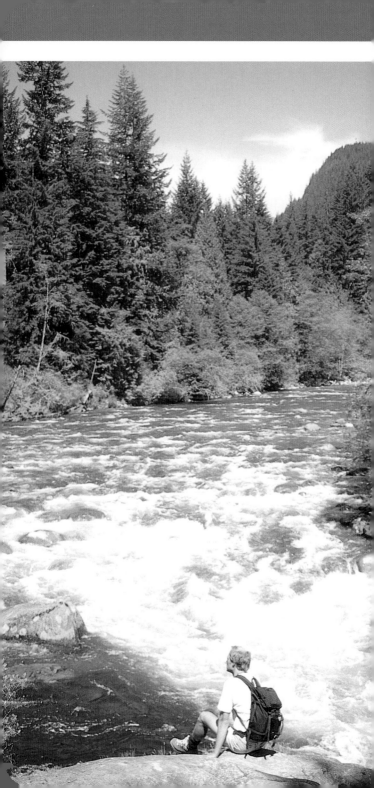

INTRODUCTION

HOW TO USE THIS BOOK

The hikes are clustered by area. At the back of the book you'll also find indexes that allow you to hunt a destination down alphabetically or according to the hike's duration, season and difficulty.

Maps

The maps that accompany the hikes in this book are meant to give an idea of the general location and direction of the trail; they are not meant as navigational aids. Topographical maps (1:50,000) can provide the best geographical detail, although trails are not always indicated. Park maps are also useful. See *Information Sources* on page 355 for more details.

Access

Unless noted, the trailheads are vehicle-accessible. (In some cases, however, such as Brandywine Meadows and Blowdown Pass, without a four-wheel drive vehicle you may have to cover a bit of extra ground on foot.) Exceptions are Mount Artaban and Widgeon Falls, which are accessible only by water, and Mount Cheam, which requires a four-wheel drive vehicle.

If access is along a forest service road, such as Cougar Mountain or High Falls Creek, where there is active logging in the area, be sure to drive with your headlights on and be especially aware of oncoming logging trucks. Weekends are usually free of such activity, but you never know.

Trailheads

Every hike starts with a trailhead. The best trailheads have signs and maps, and others will only be marked by a fluttering piece of orange tape.

Unfortunately, trailheads are often a destination for thieves. To make your vehicle less tempting, be sure to leave absolutely nothing inside. Cars have been broken into to get at a handful of parking change, a pair of sunglasses or a blanket that looked like it might be covering something more valuable.

If your vehicle is broken into, report it to the local police or RCMP. They may not be able to recover your stolen goods, but your report may result in increased police presence and fewer break-ins.

Seymour River in spring.

HIKES AND WALKS OF SOUTHWESTERN BC

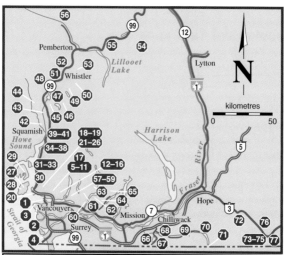

1. Stanley Park
2. Pacific Spirit Park
3. Point Grey Foreshore
4. Brunswick Point
5. Capilano Canyon
6. Goat Mountain & Ridge
7. Hanes Valley
8. Mosquito Ck Cascades
9. Lynn Creek & Forest Loop
10. Norvan Falls
11. Lynn Peak
12. Lynn Canyon & Seymour River Loop
13. Seymour River & Rice Lake Loop
14. Mount Seymour
15. Dog Mountain
16. Baden-Powell: Deep Cove to Lynn Canyon
17. Baden-Powell: Lynn Canyon to Grouse Mtn
18. Baden-Powell: Cleveland Dam to Cypress Bowl
19. Baden-Powell: Cypress Bowl to Eagle Ridge
20. Lighthouse Park
21. Cypress Falls

22. Black Mountain
23. Mount Strachan
24. Hollyburn Peak
25. Hollyburn Ridge
26. Brothers Creek Loop
27. Killarney Lake
28. Mount Gardner
29. Mount Artaban
30. St. Mark's Summit
31. The Lions
32. Howe Sound Bluffs
33. Deeks Lake
34. Petgill Lake
35. Stawamus Chief, S. Summit
36. S. Chief, C. & N. Smts.
37. Stawamus Squaw
38. Upper Shannon Falls
39. Elfin Lakes
40. Opal Cone
41. Alice Lake Prov. Park
42. Levette Lake Loop
43. Cheakamus Canyon
44. High Falls Creek
45. Garibaldi Lake
46. Panorama Ridge
47. Black Tusk
48. Brandywine Meadows
49. Cheakamus Lake

50. Russet Lake
51. Rainbow Lake
52. Cougar Mountain
53. Wedgemount Lake
54. Blowdown L. & Pass
55. Joffre Lakes
56. Tenquille Lake
57. Buntzen Lake
58. Sendero Diez Vistas
59. Eagle Ridge
60. Minnekhada Park
61. Munro & Dennett L.
62. Pitt Wildlife Loop
63. Widgeon Falls
64. Alouette Ridge
65. Gold Creek Falls
66. Vedder Ridge
67. Teapot Hill
68. Mount Cheam
69. Ford Mountain
70. Lindeman & Green-drop Lakes
71. Chilliwack River
72. Skagit River
73. Snow Camp Mountain
74. Lightning Lakes
75. Larch Plateau
76. Three Brothers Mtn.
77. Windy Joe

HIKING WITH A BRAIN

Trail Smarts

Before you ever set foot on a trail, it's worth taking a few minutes to learn something about the essentials of hiking: the gear, the clothing, trail ethics and wildlife encounters.

There's one thing that you will absolutely need no matter what your destination—your brain. Common sense will take you farther and bring you back safer than any piece of equipment or high-tech gew-gaw. It will also help you cope with another trail truism: Expect the unexpected.

First, some basic tenets. Be prepared for your chosen hike. Allow enough time to get there and back in daylight hours. Carry the 10 essentials and have a trip plan. Consult and take along a guidebook. Always tell someone where you're going. Don't hike alone. And stay on the trail.

If, despite all your best intentions, you find yourself lost, follow these suggestions from the North Shore Rescue team:

Don't panic. Maintain a positive attitude if you become lost. Being lost is not dangerous if you are prepared.

Stay where you are. Help will come, and will be there sooner if you stay in one place. If you continue moving after you are lost, you'll likely get farther away from the trail and the searchers who are trying to find you.

Do not go downhill. On mountain terrain, going down often leads to dangerous natural drainages with thick bush, steep cliffs and waterfalls.

Use signalling devices. Blow a whistle, light a fire and stay visible to help searchers find you. Don't be embarrassed or afraid to call out. Remember that animals will not be attracted to your signals.

Build or seek shelter. Protect yourself from the elements. Be as comfortable as possible but, when darkness lifts, make sure you can be seen from the air by searchers in helicopters or planes.

Be aware that it could happen to you. Bad weather, early darkness or an unexpected injury can turn an easy hike into an extended crisis. By being prepared, you'll enjoy your trip in the backcountry regardless of what nature throws at you.

Essential Gear

What you take with you will, in a large part, be determined by where you are going and for how long. A two-hour walk around Brunswick Point will not require the same gear as a seven-hour slog to The Lions.

Footwear. For two-hour walks, a good pair of walking shoes or runners will be fine. For three- to four-hour trips in terrain that's not too rugged, such as the trails at Alice Lake or Capilano Canyon, lightweight hiking boots will keep your feet happier and better protected. For longer trips or those with rough trails, good leather hiking boots with ankle support and a substantial sole are essential.

The best boots are those that fit your feet best. Boots that crowd toes or allow the foot to slide around mean trouble—blisters, bruised toenails, general bipedal agony. So choose carefully and take time to make sure the boots fit well.

Backpack. No matter where you go, it's worth taking a day-pack to tote essentials, such as water and keys. Choose a day-pack that has padding on the shoulder straps and the back and that features a waist- or hip-belt. The size is up to you, as long as it comfortably fits the 10 essentials listed below.

1. **Guidebook, map and compass.** Obviously, if you're walking somewhere like the Point Grey Foreshore, it's probably safe to forego the compass. And you likely don't need a 1:50,000 topographical map. But it's a good idea to take along this guidebook and a regional park map.

   For a backcountry hike, such as Mount Seymour or Snow Camp Mountain, carrying all three is essential, as is knowing how to use a map and compass. (There are two good books to consult: *Be Expert with Map and Compass* by Bjorn Kjellstrom, and *Mountaineering: The Freedom of the Hills*, edited by Don Graydon.)

2. **Water and food.** Bring at least 1 litre of drink no matter where you go. Physical exertion makes you sweat and you need to replenish that lost fluid or your body just won't work well. Dehydration can easily lead to cramps, fatigue and heatstroke.

   Even if you're not planning lunch on the trail, carry some quick energy food, such as chocolate bars, granola bars or dried fruit—just in case things don't go as planned.

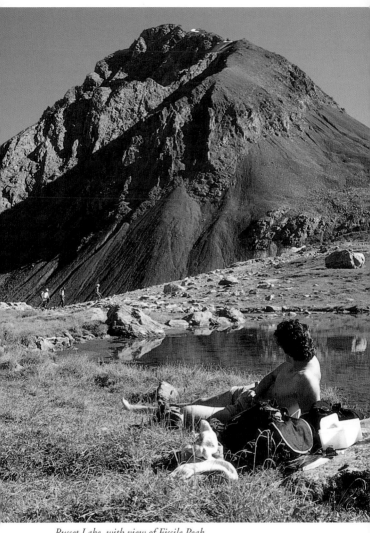

Russet Lake, with view of Fissile Peak.

3. **Extra clothes.** West Coast weather is notoriously
changeable. That means a hike that starts in warm
and sunny conditions can often finish wet and cold.
Always bring raingear—a waterproof hat, jacket and
pants—if there's even a possibility of precipitation.
For hikes at higher elevations or during cooler months
at lower elevations, bring a toque, gloves and a wool
or fleece sweater for warmth.

4. **Sunscreen, sunglasses and first-aid kit**. The sunscreen should be minimum SPF 15. The sunglasses should screen UVA and UVB rays. The first-aid kit should contain the basics: bandaids, gauze, adhesive tape, antiseptic towelettes, an elastic tensor bandage, aspirin and moleskin.

5. **Whistle.** Should you lose your way, a whistle can help let others know where you are—or help direct others who might be lost to you. The sound carries farther and lasts longer than the human voice.

6. **Pocket knife.** Infinitely useful. Once you have one you'll wonder how you ever lived without it.

7. **Flashlight or headlamp**. Even if you allowed for lots of time to return before dark, an unforeseen event such as an injury may delay you past sunset. A flashlight or headlamp will help to light the way or to illuminate whatever you're fumbling with in the dark, be it map, bandaid or pocket knife.

8. **Waterproof matches (or a lighter)**. For emergency use only. If you end up spending the night outdoors, a fire can help keep you warm and help searchers find you.

9. **Firestarter.** Suitable tinder may not be available, so take along a candle or a flattened wax carton—something that will burn easily. No matter where you are, always be careful with fire—forests have burned and alpine meadows have been scarred because of out-of-control fires.

10. **Large orange plastic bag**. It may not be high-tech, but it's multi-purpose. Such a bag can be used as a tarp or a bivouac bag to provide emergency shelter. It can also alert search crews to your location—orange is an international signal for help.

This list may seem like a lot for a dayhike, but it's really just the bare essentials. Think of it as your wilderness insurance policy.

Another essential to add is a trip itinerary. Write down where you're going, what you're wearing, what vehicle you're using to get there, who's going with you and when to expect your return. Leave it with a responsible person (who is not on the trip) so that if you fail to return, he or she can give police and rescuers crucial information. The Provincial Emergency Program provides free trip itinerary forms. Download one at www.pep.bc.ca/hazard preparedness/TripPlan.pdf.

Essential Clothing

Socks. Almost as important as the boots you wear are the socks you wear with them. Forget cotton. Cotton socks absorb sweat and create friction, which results in blisters. Instead, wear a liner sock made of polypropylene, which wicks sweat away from the foot to an outer sock, made either of wool or a polyester/wool blend. The outer sock keeps your feet warm even when damp with sweat or soaked with stream overflow or melted snow.

Gaiters. If you're a fair-weather hiker, you can probably forego this item. But if you hit the trail when it's wet or even a little snowy, gaiters will help keep your socks, boots and thus feet drier.

Shorts. Fine for summer. Nylon are best—they'll keep you cool but will dry quickly when wet.

Pants. For summer days when the weather is undecided, take along a pair of long-legged pants, preferably nylon or polyester, to keep your lower limbs warm. For the cooler days of spring, fall and winter, pants made of stretchy polyester or light fleece are best. If it's really cool, consider a thermal underlayer.

Cotton, known in outdoor circles as 'Killer Cotton,' is just no good. When wet it will cool you down, and it takes forever to dry. Leave the jeans at home.

Upper body wear. Layers are the way to go. In summer, your first layer can be a cotton tank-top or t-shirt. But bring a fleece vest or sweater in case the weather turns cool.

In spring, fall and winter, make your first layer a polyester or polypropylene top, your middle layer fleece or wool, and your outer layer a waterproof jacket. Now you can peel off or put on as the temperature demands. When you're hiking, one layer may be enough. But when you stop for lunch, you'll need more to stay warm.

Raingear. A jacket is an absolute must. Those made of Gore-Tex fabrics are best, since they'll repel the rain and still breathe. Laminated nylon or other plasticized raingear does not allow air to circulate, so although it will keep the rain off, you'll sweat like mad and end up soaked to the skin with condensation and perspiration.

Hat. In summer, a wide-brimmed hat or baseball cap will help keep the sun off your face and out of your eyes. In spring, fall or winter, a toque of fleece or wool can keep you warm. (Remember, up to 50 percent of body heat is lost through the head.)

Gloves. Fleece or wool is fine. Gloves are better than mitts.

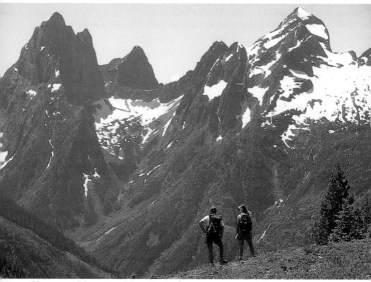

Hozameen Mountain, Manning Park.

PEEING IN THE WOODS

Yes, it is not the stuff of which polite conversations are made. But, somewhere, sometime, along the trail you're going to feel the need to relieve your bladder or bowels. If toilets are nearby, you're in luck. Otherwise, you're going to have to improvise in a way that will have the least impact possible on the surroundings. (Anyone who has come across disgusting wads of used toilet paper on the trail will appreciate this advice.)

The basic rule is to do your business at least 45 metres away from any stream, lake or other body of water. If you're dealing with a bowel movement, be sure to dig a shallow hole in the soil before, and bury the deposit afterward. Pack used toilet paper into a plastic bag and carry it out with the rest of your garbage.

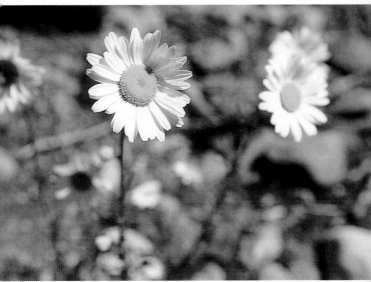

Daisies, Skagit River.

TRAIL ETHICS

Stay on the trail. Trails are constructed for reasons. They create easier access into an area. And they protect the area through which they pass from mass trampling and the destruction that results.

For those reasons, stick to the trail. Do not take erosion-causing shortcuts on switchbacks, do not trample alpine meadows to avoid a mud puddle or two, and do not walk alongside constructed stairs.

Pack out all your garbage. Do not leave behind anything you brought with you. Not only is garbage an unpleasant surprise for the next hiker, but it attracts animals, which can be potential nuisances—such as pack rats—or potential hazards—such as black bears.

Don't pick the daisies. Or any other wildflowers or plants. Don't dig up shrubs or carry off rocks or any items with heritage significance. In essence, don't take anything with you that you didn't bring in. You know, follow the famous hiker's credo: Take only photographs; leave nothing but footprints.

ENCOUNTERS WITH WILDLIFE

Flying bugs

These bugs are the forms of wildlife you're most likely to encounter on the trail. In summer, mosquitoes, no-see-ums, blackflies and deerflies can make a dayhike seem like one of the rings of hell in Dante's *Inferno*. Aside from hermetically sealing yourself in mosquito netting, your only defence is bug spray. Some people swear by sprays that contain a substance called DEET (also known as N, N-diethyl-metatoluamide), but be aware that this stuff is potent enough to dissolve plastic, paint and some synthetic fabrics.

Ticks

These little blood-sucking insects are the hiker's other big worry. They can pass on the nasty bacteria that cause Lyme disease and Rocky Mountain spotted fever, among other illnesses. The worst time for ticks is April, May or June but they can be around at any time of year.

Ticks are little sesame seed-sized creatures that can drop onto your head from an overhead branch or be picked up when walking along a brush-lined trail. They then look for some warm furry part in which to sink their pincer-like jaws. Check your body regularly for the little cretins, especially such parts as armpits, groin, head and back. Use your fingers as well as your eyes to ferret out any unusual bumps in the skin.

If you do find a tick on your body, resist the initial impulse to just rip its little body out. A tick must be removed carefully. If its body is crushed while you're trying to remove it, the contents of its gut—with any insidious bacteria—can be transmitted to your body.

It's best to have a doctor remove the tick as soon as possible. If that's not feasible, you can do it yourself using tick pliers. Grasp the tick's body and gently pull it out taking care not to squish it. Put the tick in a plastic bag or a vial with some damp cotton or grass and make sure that it goes to the Centres for Disease Control laboratories for testing.

These days, it's standard for anyone who has been bitten by a tick to start on a prophylactic program of antibiotics, just in case the tick was carrying the borreolosis bacteria responsible for Lyme disease. Although Lyme disease won't kill you, it is debilitating and painful and stays with you for the rest of your life.

Bears

I have yet to meet a hiker who does not have bears on the brain. Yes, all bears are potentially dangerous. Yes, bears have killed people. And yes, bears have seriously injured people. But such attacks are rare. In BC, between 1978 and 1996, bears fatally mauled 14 people. Every year on average, bears injure seven people. (By comparison, almost 1000 bears are killed because of human/bear conflicts each year.) You can keep those numbers from climbing by learning more about bears before you go hiking, and by practising bear-aware tactics on the trail.

Most of southwestern BC is the realm of the black bear (*Ursus americanus*). Black bears live wherever there is adequate food and cover (brush or forest). In the Lower Mainland, black bears are often seen on the slopes of the North Shore mountains. And they are occasionally seen in Maple Ridge, Pitt Meadows and Surrey.

Grizzly bears (*Ursus arctos*) have been seen as far south as Squamish, but they are more likely to hang out where there are fewer people. The Pemberton–Whistler area is griz territory.

Pick up a book such as *Bear Attacks: Their Causes and Avoidance* by Stephen Herrero, a University of Calgary professor who is probably North America's pre-eminent bear expert, and learn more about bears. Knowing such things as what bears eat at which time of year, and what are the signs of bears, lessens the likelihood of an encounter.

Here are some hints for the trail:

Make noise. Talk, sing, shout or clap your hands. But forget about bear-bells. 'In Glacier National Park,' says BC Wildlife Branch bear biologist Tony Hamilton, 'it's like ringing a dinner bell. The bears there have clued in that the bells mean food is coming. The sound of the human voice is far better.'

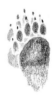

Don't hike alone. Herrero found that small parties of one or two people were attacked more often than larger groups.

If you do encounter a bear on the trail, the first thing to do is determine whether the bear is a black or a grizzly. And whether an impending attack is defensive or predatory.

If you have startled a bear, come too near to a mother with cubs or are seen as too close to a food source, the bear likely sees you as a threat. If you're far enough away, the bear will let you know that it's agitated by huffing or hissing, turning broadside, urinating, rising on its hind legs or circling around to get a better scent.

In those cases, you can minimize your threat by backing away slowly while waving your arms slowly and talking in a calm voice. Never turn and run, as that will only trigger a bear's innate predator response.

If you're too close for the bear's comfort, it will likely charge. What you do next is still the stuff of controversy. Most experts agree that if the bear charging you is a grizzly responding to a perceived threat, you should drop to the ground, cover your head and neck, and roll yourself into a tight ball to protect your internal organs. Even if the grizzly begins chewing on you, stay quiet. Never fight back.

If, however, the bear attacking is a black bear, opinion is divided. Some experts, such as Herrero, advise fighting back only if the attack is predatory. Others, such as Hamilton, advise fighting back no matter what the situation. 'The reasoning is,' he says, 'that among black bears, defensive attacks are rare. And, given that most adults in BC could be a formidable opponent to most black bears in BC, fighting back is your best response.'

Both experts agree that fighting back is the appropriate response in one particular situation—when a bear sees you not as a threat, but as a potential meal. 'Those circumstances are extremely rare,' says Hamilton, 'But with a predatory attack, you want to give the opposite message to a bear—that you're not just going to lie down and be dinner.'

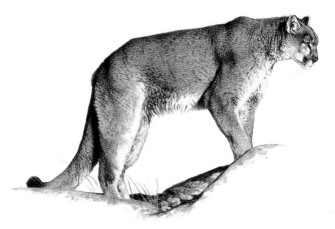

Cougars

Although it's rare to see cougars on the trail, it does happen. Children are more likely to be the target of a cougar attack, but incidents in the last few years have involved adults.

As with bears, your best defence is to make noise on the trail. Given half a chance, most cougars would rather keep any company than that of human beings.

If, however, you do encounter a cougar, it's recommended that you make yourself out to be as big and bad as you possibly can. Wave your arms and make a hellish amount of noise, all the time backing up slowly. **Never** turn and run. It will only trigger the animal's innate predatory response.

If the animal approaches, throw rocks or sticks or whatever is on hand. Again, you want to impress upon the cougar that you will not be an easy meal.

ABOUT SOUTHWESTERN BC

People love southwestern BC for its natural assets—the mountains, glaciers, forests, meadows, rivers, lakes and ocean. These are the same elements that draw hikers to the trail. And if you're like me, you'll find that the more trails you hike, the more mountains you scramble up, the more meadows you traverse, the more forests you walk through, the more you want to know about them.

Whether it's the thin lines etched on rock by an ancient glacier, the towering splendour of a 60-metre-tall Douglas fir, the tiny perfection of a rein orchid, the cheeky brashness of a gray jay or the inexplicable way that rain seems to come from nowhere, something at some time will pique your interest and make you wonder why.

Below are a few tidbits of the natural history of southwestern BC and some recommendations on where to find out more.

Geology

When you are hiking any of the trails in this book, you will essentially be in one of three geographic units: the Coast Mountains, the Fraser Lowland or the Cascade Mountains.

The North Shore mountains and all points north lie within the Coast Mountain Range. They are among the youngest rocks in the province, having been born of molten rock far below the Earth's surface about 90 to 100 million years ago. Underground rock was eventually lifted by various tectonic forces and eroded by rivers and streams. Later, when sheets of ice surged as far south as Seattle, the rock was sculpted by glaciers.

Granitic rock is the stuff of which most of the Coast Mountains are made. The Stawamus Chief is a single, stunning example of such rock, made up mostly of grey quartz, white plagioclase and pink potassium feldspar.

Other Coast Range rock is even younger, having spewed forth as lava as recently as 8000 years ago from a chain of volcanoes that includes Mount Garibaldi. (Garibaldi itself is estimated to have been created 10,000 to 15,000 years ago, but other volcanoes in the same chain have erupted more recently.)

The Fraser Lowland is a roughly triangular depression between the Coast Mountains and the Cascade Mountains. One side of the triangle runs from Agassiz northwest to Stanley Park; another runs from Agassiz southwest to Bellingham in the US.

With the exception of low mountains such as Sumas and

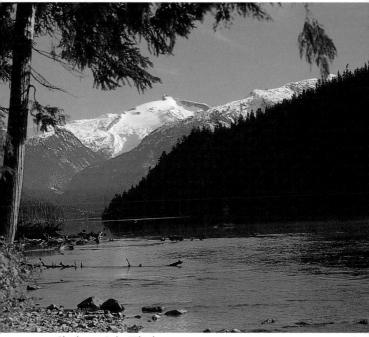
Cheakamus Lake, Whistler area.

Burnaby, the land ranges from flat prairie to rolling hills. The rock here is sedimentary, deposited by rivers and streams starting about 70 million years ago. The exposed cliffs of the Point Grey Foreshore are good places to see such stuff in cross-section.

The peaks of Mount Cheam and Ford Mountain lie within the Cascade Mountain Range, as do Vedder Ridge, Teapot Hill, Lindeman and Greendrop Lakes. Within such a relatively small geographic area, the rock ranges from 30 to 350 million years in age.

At some of the highest elevations of the Cheam Range, fossils of ancient sea creatures have been found, dating the rock up to 350 million years old, when an inland sea inundated land that was much lower than today.

But most of the peaks in the Chilliwack area originated about 30 million years ago when magma bubbled up below the surface, hardened, then was eroded by water and sculpted by ice into today's mountains. The area has also seen volcanic activity, most notably from nearby Mount Baker. The Cascades lie along the same 'Ring of fire' that includes Mounts Garibaldi and Meager of the Coast Range.

Flora

The range of plant life in BC is so vast and complex that it's difficult to know where to begin. And if you look to ecosections, biogeoclimatic zones, site associations and other ways that scientists attempt to give some order to the plant universe, it can seem bewildering. But really it's just a matter of terminology.

Using something called Ecosystem Classification, the province has been divided into five levels on the basis of climate and landforms. The system starts with ecodomains and ecodivisions—which, in essence, put BC in a global context—then makes further distinctions to come up with eight ecoprovinces, even more ecoregions and 72 ecosections.

But, because the type of vegetation within an ecosection varies according to elevation and climate, there's also a system of biogeoclimatic zones, sort of like chapters in a book. In BC, there are 14 such zones. The hikes in this book cover terrain that lies in six zones: Coastal Western Hemlock, Mountain Hemlock, Alpine Tundra, Engelmann Spruce-Subalpine Fir, Montane Spruce and Interior Douglas Fir.

Coastal Western Hemlock. This zone occurs at low to middle elevations—sea level to 1000 metres—on the coast. Characterized by cool summers and mild winters, it is the wettest biogeoclimatic zone in BC and can get as much as 5 metres of rain per year.

Western hemlock is the most common tree species, often accompanied by amabilis fir. Western red cedar and yellow cedar are common but less frequent as elevation increases. Sitka spruce, western white pine, Pacific yew, red alder and broadleaf maple also make up the forest.

In the forest understorey are shrubs such as vine maple, salmonberry, blueberry, huckleberry, salal and Oregon grape, as well as a variety of ferns, mosses and lichens.

Mountain Hemlock. This zone occurs on the coast at elevations between 900 and 1800 metres and is characterized by short, cool summers and long, cool, wet winters with heavy snowcover for several months.

Mountain hemlock, amabilis fir and yellow cedar are the most common tree species. Forests tend to be continuous only at the lower elevations. As elevation increases, the forest thins into parkland, and several species of mountain heather occur. The predominant shrubs in the acidic soils found here are blueberry, huckleberry, copperbush, azalea and rhododendron.

This zone also features subalpine meadows, resplendent in summer with such wildflowers as yellow glacier lilies,

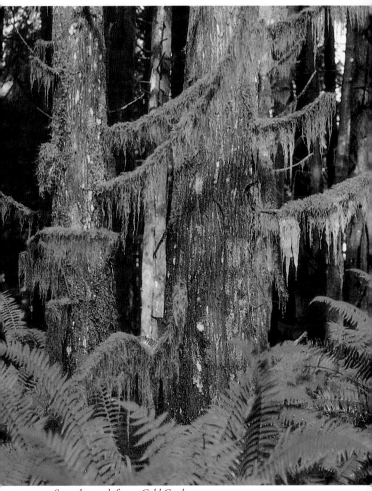

Second-growth forest, Gold Creek.

blue lupines, red Indian paintbrush and white Sitka valerian.

Alpine Tundra. This zone starts at above 1500 metres on the windward side of mountains, and above 1800 metres on the leeward side. The climate is cold, windy and snowy, and is characterized by a short growing season during a brief frost-free period. Mean annual temperatures range from -4° to 0°C. Most of the annual precipitation falls as snow.

Trees are only found at the lowest elevations and include subalpine fir, Engelmann spruce, white spruce, mountain hemlock and whitebark pine. Often trees are gnarled, wizened krummholz trees—*krummholz* means 'crooked' in German. Alpine vegetation is dominated by shrubs, herbs, mosses and lichens.

Tiny alpine wildflowers occur—bonsai versions of their brothers and sisters at lower elevations, cropped by the cold, wind and snow.

Engelmann Spruce-Subalpine fir and **Montane Spruce**. These zones occurs at higher elevations—from 1200 to 2200 metres—in the southern interior; Manning Provincial Park is an example. The climate is drier, with warmer summers, colder winters and a short growing season.

The most common tree species found are Engelmann spruce and subalpine fir, although lodgepole pine, amabilis fir and the occasional Douglas fir or western hemlock can be found as well.

In the understorey are shrubs, grasses, dryland mosses and lichen. Near the treeline, beautiful, often lush wildflowers mingle with the sparsely spaced trees.

Interior Douglas fir. This zone occurs at lower to middle elevations—300 to 1300 metres—in the southern interior of the province, from parts of Manning Provincial Park to north of Williams Lake. Climate is drier and colder than on the coast.

The most common tree species found is Douglas fir, which grows to shorter heights and smaller girths than on the coast. Lodgepole pine, ponderosa pine, aspen, birch and western yew are also present. In areas that receive more moisture, western red cedar and western white pine are also found.

The understorey is predominantly pinegrass, with wildflowers such as yarrow, aster, wild strawberry and pussytoes.

These six zones can be further broken down to site associations—too specific to go into detail here—that distinguish the predominant vegetation according to elevation and rain or snowfall.

What's important to remember is that describing a place in such terms is not merely a pedantic scientific exercise. It also plays a pivotal role in determining which areas will be designated as parks. Under the Protected Areas Strategy, the province has promised to protect 12 percent of the land base from development. Although it would be easier to designate hectares of rock and ice—in which resource extraction industries such as logging have little interest—the 12 percent must also include undisturbed areas such as low-elevation old-growth forests, which are rare in some parts of the province.

Fauna

More than 1000 animal species inhabit the province of BC (as well as 42,000 insect species). Some, such as northern spotted owls, mountain beavers and wolverines, are rarely seen; others, such as northwestern crows, gray jays and Douglas squirrels, seem to be everywhere.

Among the mammals you're more likely to see when hiking are black bear, black-tailed deer, mule deer, beaver, raccoon, spotted skunk, striped skunk, rabbit, hoary marmot, pika, northwestern chipmunk, Douglas squirrel, northern flying squirrel and deer mouse.

Among the birds you're likely to see are great blue heron, bald eagle, red-tailed hawk, blue grouse, barred owl, downy woodpecker, hairy woodpecker, pileated woodpecker, Steller's jay, gray jay, Clark's nutcracker, northwestern crow, raven, black-capped chickadee, American dipper, Townsend's warbler, dark-eyed junco, house sparrow and rufous hummingbird.

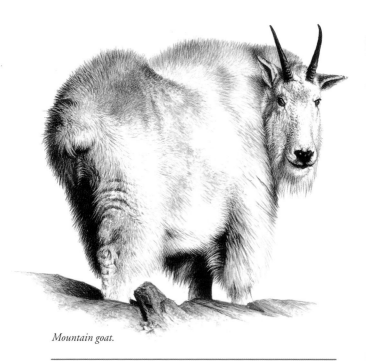

Mountain goat.

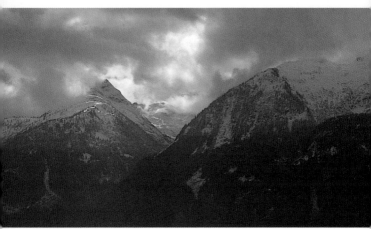
Tantalus Range, viewed from Cheakamus Canyon.

Weather

In much the same way as the Inuit have many words for snow, Lower Mainlanders distinguish the varieties of rain: from drizzle to downpour, from spit to showers.

Here on the proverbial 'wet coast,' the amount of rainfall varies from less than 1000 millimetres a year on the flatlands near Boundary Bay, to more than 3000 millimetres annually in the upper reaches of the North Shore mountains.

Blame it on the ocean, and to some extent, the mountains—the same two elements that lure Lower Mainlanders out of doors. We live in a maritime climate, where westerly winds bring moisture-laden air to our doorstep. Where there are mountains, the clouds drop that moisture more quickly.

Still, it's not all doom and gloom. Southwestern BC also averages about 2000 hours of sunshine per year. And the average winter temperature hovers around 5°C while elsewhere in the country, people shiver to -20°C.

FURTHER READING

Further information on the flora and fauna, geology and weather of southwestern BC is available in the following books, fully listed in the Selected Bibliography on page 354:

British Columbia, A Natural History
Field Guide to the Birds of North America
Garibaldi Geology
Mammals of the Canadian Wild
Plants of Coast British Columbia
Plants of Southern Interior British Columbia
Vancouver Geology.

VANCOUVER AREA

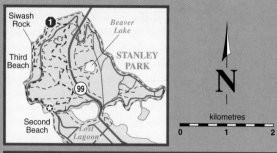

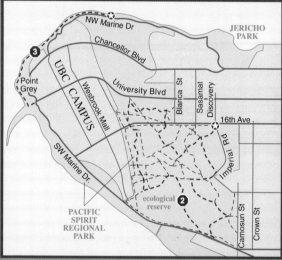

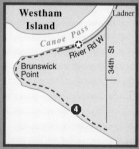

1 Stanley Park, p. 32
2 Pacific Spirit Park, p. 37
3 Point Grey Foreshore, p. 41
4 Brunswick Point, p. 44

1 STANLEY PARK

Distance: 7 km	Season: Year-round
Elevation gain: Minimal	Trail map: Page 31
High point: 50 m	
Time needed: 2 hours	
Rating: Easy	

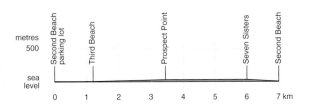

EVERY DAY, THOUSANDS OF PEOPLE WALK, jog, cycle or rollerblade the concrete seawall that encircles Stanley Park. Few leave that seaside periphery to explore the system of trails within the park's 405 hectares. But what those trails lead to—stunning old-growth trees, gorgeous ocean views and tranquillity—makes them 'must-walk' destinations.

Our route starts at Second Beach. Head into the forest on the far side of the roadway—trails connect from either end of the parking lots. Turn left at the first trail that crosses your path and head north. The Rawlings Trail shadows the road for about a kilometre, ambling past wondrous western red cedars and equally tall broadleaf maples, in winter recognizable by their leafless limbs covered with elaborate sweaters of moss and ferns.

After you've passed the Ferguson Point Teahouse and the turnoff to Third Beach, a trail cuts across your path. Turn left and follow Tatlow Walk across the road and down to where it emerges north of the Third Beach concession. Here the trail forks into 4 separate paths. Go right—the signs point to Prospect Point and the Hollow Tree—for a little side-trip.

Only 150 metres upslope is the biggest cedar in the park. It's not the tree's 45-metre height that's amazing, although the sight of its red-riveted bark towering against a blue sky is awesome. It's the girth: almost 14 metres, about as thick around as the Point Atkinson Lighthouse.

Much larger trees once dominated the park—as they once dominated all of the city—but selective logging during the

Western red cedar.

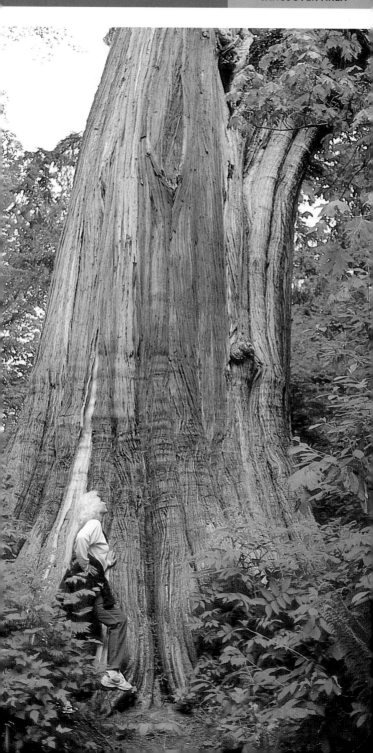

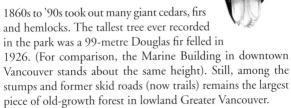

Although increasingly rare in many areas, bald eagles are seen in Stanley Park.

1860s to '90s took out many giant cedars, firs and hemlocks. The tallest tree ever recorded in the park was a 99-metre Douglas fir felled in 1926. (For comparison, the Marine Building in downtown Vancouver stands about the same height). Still, among the stumps and former skid roads (now trails) remains the largest piece of old-growth forest in lowland Greater Vancouver.

Retrace your steps to the fork in the trail and go right on Merilees Trail. A mere 100 metres farther is another big tree, this time a Sitka spruce almost 46 metres high. A slight bend in its slender trunk makes it look almost too delicate to hold such weight upright, but it has been doing so for hundreds of years.

At the next trail intersection, go left to a viewpoint of English Bay, artfully framed by cedar, hemlock and salal—something you don't see from the seawall, although you're now directly above it. Follow the trail as it drops down and, at the clearing, bear left to the viewpoint at Siwash Rock.

The Coast Salish people know this rock as Slahkayulsh, or 'He who is standing up.' The name refers to a man famed both as a warrior and a father. By Pauline Johnson's 1911 account in *Legends of Vancouver*, the man was swimming in the narrows—according to tradition—while his wife gave birth to their child within the forests at Prospect Point.

> It was the law that he must be clean, spotlessly clean, so that when his child looked out upon the world it would have the chance to live its own life clean.

While he swam, a canoe paddled up, bearing four giant men who were the agents of Sagalie Tyee (God). They told him to move out of their way, but the father-to-be said he could not stop swimming nor go ashore nor do anything that would interfere with the purity of his coming child's life. The four men were dumbstruck; no man had ever defied them before. While they talked about what to do, the faint cry of a child emanated from the forest. The swimmer ceased his stroke.

> "Because you have placed that child's future before all things," said the tallest of the four men, "you shall never die, but shall

Siwash Rock.

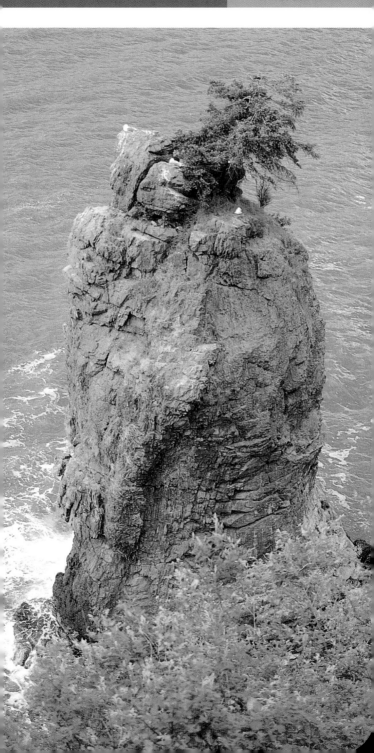

stand through all the thousands of years to come where all eyes can see you...as an indestructible monument to Clean Fatherhood."

As the feet of the young chief touched the shore, he was transformed into stone. And that is the story of how Siwash Rock came to be.

Continue along the clifftop trail for more views of the ocean and the North Shore mountains. After 10 minutes, look up, way up, for a big bare snag. At 72 metres tall, this now-dead Douglas fir is the second tallest in Stanley Park. Another dead fir near Pipeline Road peaks out at 76.2 metres. Bald eagles, such as the two juveniles I saw perched on the highest branches, favour such giants.

Many large living trees still grow alongside Merilees Trail. The tallest hemlock in the park stands 50 metres high near the next junction (where you go right to join an upper trail), but it can be tough to see because all of the other trees here also seem to be in the 50- to 60-metre range.

Merilees Trail ends at the roadway. Cross the road and follow the trail on the right. Ten minutes farther is an intersection; continue straight ahead to the next junction and go right. At the next junction stands a 53-metre high cottonwood. Go left to pick up Thompson Trail. Within minutes, a big, beautiful candelabra cedar stands before you. At times, sunlight hits the tree to make it appear like a beacon in the forest darkness. The next 200 metres of trail are lined by many big beautiful cedars, including one cluster known as the Three Graces because of the three separate but close-knit trunks.

If it hasn't hit you already, consider this: Where else in the world could you see such a forest in the downtown of a major city? Traffic noise from the causeway builds as you near the next intersection, where you'll bear right to follow Bridle Path but only as far as the next junction. (The pedestrian crossing over the causeway is here.)

Go right. Then, 50 metres later, go left on Squirrel Trail. At its end, continue south to Tatlow Walk. Go left and amble alongside one of the wettest sections of the forest—a virtual cedar heaven. The park's tallest cedar (56.2 metres) resides here.

At the next intersection are the Seven Sisters, or as they're now cheekily known, the Seven Stumps. The grove of giant Douglas firs and western red cedars were lopped down in 1951. Fifty metres beyond is a four-pronged junction. Go right onto the Bridle Path Trail, which you can follow back to Second Beach. The seawall may never look the same again.

PACIFIC SPIRIT REGIONAL PARK

2

Distance: Up to 10 km return

Elevation gain: Minimal

High Point: 50 m

Time needed: Up to 3 hours

Rating: Easy

Season: Year-round

Topographical map:
North Vancouver 92G/6

Trail map: Page 31

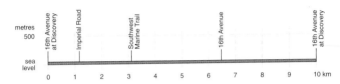

WITH MORE THAN 50 KILOMETRES OF trails within more than 750 hectares of forest and foreshore, Pacific Spirit Regional Park is a winter walker's dream—especially on those days when it's pouring rain but you just have to get out.

The parks department of the Greater Vancouver Regional District (GVRD) maintains the trails, and provides a detailed map to make navigating the forested maze easy. You can design your own hike and explore without fear of getting lost on the way. (Just remember to allow enough daylight hours.)

Our designer hike starts on the southwest corner of 16th and Discovery, where Huckleberry Trail (#11) leads into the trees. At this point, you're on a trail set aside for foot traffic only—despite the occasional mountain bike tread mushed into the mud.

Continue on to where the trail intersects with Top Trail (#25) and turn left. For the next few minutes, you'll wander along the edges of an important wetland: the headwaters of Musqueam Creek and home to lots of amphibians. You may also see the concrete foundations of a radio antenna once used by the Northwest Telephone Company.

Eventually, the trail spills onto Imperial Road. Turn right and walk on the roadside for about 100 metres then head back into the forest again, this time along Imperial Trail (#12). Now, for the first time, you're on a multi-use trail, where walkers mingle with cyclists and horseback riders. Walkers tend to be the users who move out of the way to let bikes and horses by. The rules of the road for everyone are simple: Be aware and be courteous.

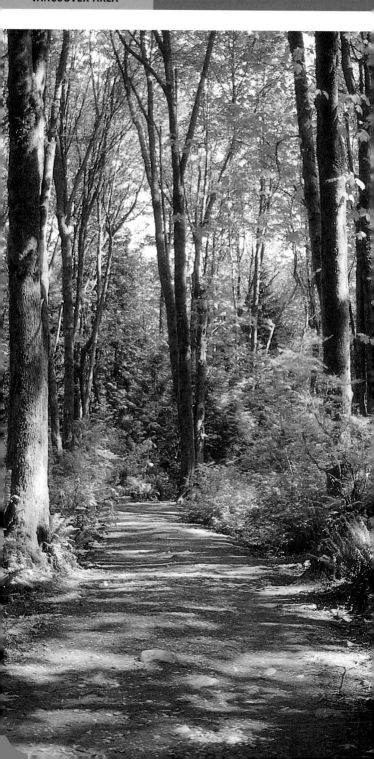

In winter, Musqueam Creek—one of the very few old streams in Vancouver never filled in or otherwise altered—tinkles alongside as you follow Imperial into the heart of the park. In summer, the creek tends to dry up and more closely resemble a damp ditch. But now a project is under way that may add water to both Musqueam and Cutthroat creeks during summer low flow, in order to help fish survive in both streams.

Where the creek takes a sharp left to shadow Hemlock Trail (#9), so will you. Here, the path meanders through second-growth forest that is punctuated by numerous stumps—red cedar and Douglas fir—which were logged in the 1880s and '90s. Hemlock, red cedar, vine and broadleaf maple now replace the former giants.

A few minutes farther, the trail joins up with Sasamat Trail (#22). Continue straight ahead (south) for another few minutes until the intersection with Clinton Trail (#3). The Clinton family once ran a stable in this clearing: Charles Clinton opened the Point Grey Riding Club in 1927; he and son Alf operated it until 1962.

From here, the trail drops downhill to cross a peaceful gladed portion of Musqueam Creek before emerging to a clearing adjacent to SW Marine Drive.

Head right to pick up Salish Trail (#21). Traffic noise fades as you follow the trail along the eastern boundaries of Ecological Reserve #74. Eighty-nine hectares of forest were set aside in 1975 to preserve a second-growth forest ecosystem close to the university. Access to the reserve is controlled; special permits are available for research and educational projects only.

After 30 minutes or so of walking through one of the park's quieter sections, Salish meets up again with Imperial Trail. Go left and straight along Imperial until it forks. Then, bear left to follow along the northwestern boundary of the ecological reserve. A small bridge crosses Cutthroat Creek, home to an endangered strain of cutthroat trout (about the size of a finger, they're original stock). Recently, there have been problems with mountain bikers and dogs taking shortcuts through the tiny creek, causing erosion and silting. Don't do it.

A few minutes later, you pass the junction with Iron Knee Trail. About 75 metres farther, the trail meets up with Sword Fern Trail (#24)—one of the longest trails in the park. Head right along this walking-only path and follow it for a kilometre or so as it meanders past old monster stumps and second-growth, hopping across several east-west multi-use trails.

Pastoral woodland trail, Pacific Spirit Park.

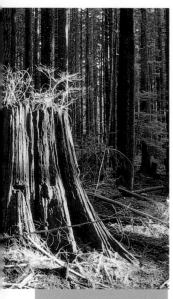

Ramble through the second-growth forests, crossing over ancient creeks, passing remnant stumps of forest giants and skirting the periphery of an ecological reserve—all within three hours.

The section of trail just before it meets up with Salish again is often 100 metres or so of unrelenting puddles, mud and ooze. At the junction, bear left and emerge onto 16th Avenue. If you've had enough, simply go right and return to the starting point along the raised Sherry Sakamoto Trail (#30), named after the woman who won the 1989 park-naming contest.

If you still have a yearning to wander, cross 16th Avenue and head into the more deciduous woods along Salish. Bear right where the trail forks and follow it past Heron Trail to the Lily of the Valley Trail (#13), designated for walkers only. Just after the path crosses the Cleveland Trail, you'll encounter the biggest stumps in the park—huge western red cedar, some as large as 7 metres in girth.

A local artist, inspired by the cedars, began to carve one of the stumps. But GVRD Parks had complaints from park visitors who were concerned about natural values giving way to a gnome garden, so they asked the artist to refrain. Parts of the stump figure have since been vandalized.

When the path meets the Salal Trail (#20), turn right and head back to 16th and across the road. Here again, you may head back to the starting point. But, if you want just a few more minutes of forested bliss, follow Salal back into the trees. A left turn on Cleveland Trail, a quick left jig on Nature Trail (#15), and a right onto Deer Fern Trail (#5) will bring you to a stand of almost all Douglas fir. A large fire swept through here in the 1920s, after the area was logged. The hard-packed soil left behind is what Douglas firs prefer to grow in.

Where Deer Fern ends, turn left to find yourself once again on Huckleberry Trail, which you need only follow for a few minutes farther, straight out to where you started.

POINT GREY FORESHORE

3

Distance: 6–13 km	Rating: Easy
Elevation gain: Minimal	Season: Year-round
High point: Sea level	Topographical map:
Time needed: 2–5 hours	North Vancouver 92G/6
	Trail map: Page 31
Note: Bring binoculars.	

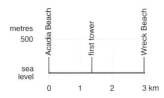

metres
500

Acadia Beach

first tower

Wreck Beach

sea
level

0   1   2   3 km

DURING THE DARKEST DAYS OF WINTER, getting out for a long walk calls for spontaneity. When the downpours let up and enough daylight still remains, you want to get to a trailhead as soon as possible.

For those people living on the North Shore, or in outlying areas near to a park, it's a quick trip. But for the thousands of people who live in the city, it's not quite so simple to get away from the buildings and the concrete for a walk on the wild side. Unless, of course, you head for Point Grey.

Here, where the shoreline is your trail, natural beauty abounds in the form of wildlife, ocean vistas and geological points of interest. Your starting point is Acadia Beach, located off NW Marine Drive at the westernmost end of Spanish Banks. The walk starts from the parking lot just where the road begins its long uphill haul to UBC.

Follow the trail down towards the beach to be greeted by views of English Bay, with Bowen Island stretching out in front and the mountains of the Sunshine Coast peeking from behind. The much smaller Passage Island lies in the middle of the bay, just off Eagle Harbour in West Vancouver.

> Just off shore, flocks of sea ducks, such as surf scoters, buffleheads and goldeneyes, dive in search of mussels and other marine delicacies. Also bobbing among the waves are harbour seals—lots of them.

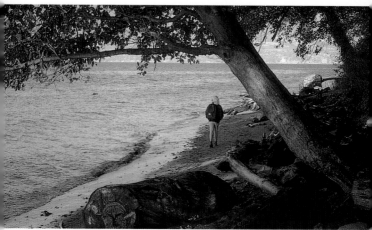

Point Grey Foreshore.

In summer, this point marks the start of clothing-optional territory (it's a nude beach). But in winter, the only bare limbs are those of the surrounding trees and shrubs—maple, alder and thimbleberry among them. The path crosses a simple yet slippery bridge and not much farther forks. Go right.

From here, the beach is your footpath: on the sandy sections, the walking is easy; on the rocky parts, watch your footing on the often slimy or frosty rocks. It's not unusual to see the most seals in these waters during December, January and February, says Jeff Marliave, a marine biologist at The Vancouver Aquarium. Nobody really knows why. Winter, it seems, is the least understood season when it comes to seals. But marine biologists have observed that in winter seals spend more time in the water than on shore. In summer, seals can often be seen lolling around on everything from shoreside rocks to log booms to boat docks.

Use your binoculars to watch the seals' offshore antics, and look for the occasional eagle perching on the few cedars growing among the leafless deciduous trees.

The eroded cliffsides show the geological nature of the area—layer upon layer of mud, sand and clay carried from the Fraser River and deposited on the shores of Point Grey. Years ago, when the long Iona jetty was built, currents and deposition patterns changed and erosion scraped away the beaches and cliffs here. Since then, work has been done to control the ocean-generated erosion, but the annual monsoons still take a toll, as evidenced by the exposed tree roots and downed trees that you must hop over.

After 30 minutes or so of relaxed walking, comes Tower Beach and the first of two namesake towers that housed searchlights as part of the Point Grey battery built during the early 1940s. Higher up the slope are the remnants of the gun emplacements, shell lockers and underground magazines, which were to be the first line of defence against the attacks by the Japanese then felt to be imminent. (The only boat ever intercepted was an anchored freighter struck by a ricocheting warning shot, which had been fired at a fish-packing boat oblivious to the wartime crisis.)

This point also marks the first of the trails that head upslope and loop back to the parking lot. The trail behind the first tower rises steeply to emerge where Marine Drive intersects with Chancellor Boulevard.

We, however, will continue along the beach past the first of the berms of smooth rounded river stones brought in to control erosion of the cliffs behind the Museum of Anthropology. Heading towards the second tower, the views change. On clear days you can see across Georgia Strait to the blue outlines of Vancouver Island; on cloudy days, you can pretend it's the limitless horizon of the Pacific Ocean.

Had you been looking in this direction in say, 1791, you might have seen the Spanish schooner *Santa Saturnina* anchored offshore. On board were Lieutenant José María Narváez and crew, who mistakenly believed that the headland in the near distance was an island (on the charts, Point Grey is referred to as 'Isla de Langara'). The Spanish did not land, but some of the Musqueam people paddled out to trade meat, vegetables and firewood for sheets of copper and pieces of iron. A year later, Captain George Vancouver sailed by on his way to explore Burrard Inlet.

Rounding the corner after the second tower, you catch sight of the light beacon at the end of the North Arm breakwater off Wreck Beach. Another 150 metres farther is Trail Four, on which you can ascend to Marine Drive near the Museum of Anthropology, and head back to the lot for a round trip of about two hours.

But we will continue along the rocky shore. Rounding the point, you'll get the first glimpse of Wreck Beach, marked by a couple of tattered banners flying from a forest of poles—logs that have been propped upright by beachgoers over the years. From here, you can ascend the steepness of Trail Six to Marine Drive and a 45-minute walk back to the parking lot. Or poke farther along a slopeside-trail to a section of Old Marine Drive. Or dawdle back along the shore you came through on.

4 BRUNSWICK POINT

Distance: 7–14 km return	Rating: Easy
Elevation gain: None	Season: Year-round
High point: Sea level	Topographical map:
Time needed: 2 hours	New Westminster 92G/3
	Trail map: Page 31

Note: Bring binoculars to watch the birds.

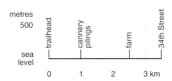

metres 500 — trailhead — cannery pilings — farm — 34th Street

sea level

0   1   2   3 km

THE DYKES THAT PROTECT THE LOWLANDS of the Lower Mainland from flooding also serve an important recreational function—they're great byways for walkers, cyclists and horseback riders.

Many dyke systems, however, abut suburban backyards, and walking them hardly creates the feeling of getting away from it all. The dyke that hugs Brunswick Point is a happy exception.

The best place to start this easy hike is from the westernmost portion of River Road in Ladner, past the turnoff for the Reifel Migratory Bird Sanctuary. At 34th Street, there are a few spots for parking, either alongside or atop the dyke. Farther west, there are a few more.

As you gain the gravel dyketop at 34th Street, views of Canoe Pass and Westham Island greet you. Harbour seals cruise the outflow currents of the river, only their dog-like heads visible above the flat brown waters. Farther ahead, old pilings bop and sway to an estuarine beat.

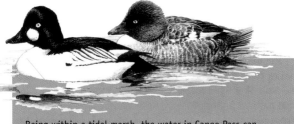

Being within a tidal marsh, the water in Canoe Pass can really scoot at times of changing tides. Ducks, gulls and other waterfowl zip past as if on some long liquid conveyor belt out to sea.

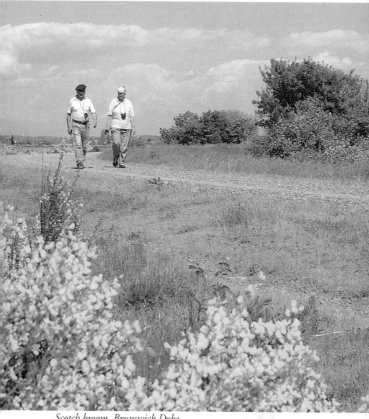

Scotch broom, Brunswick Dyke.

As River Road ends below, the dyke passes an old farmstead. Only one building now remains, its moss-covered roof folded inward to dilapidation.

Just beyond are the pilings that mark the site of the old Brunswick Cannery, one of 14 canneries in Delta. In the 1870s and 1880s, a wider and deeper Canoe Pass teemed with both salmon and canneries. It is said that as many as 75,000 salmon were caught on a single night. The canning industry boomed along until years of successive flooding in the 1890s helped to silt in Canoe Pass, and a cannery set up at Point Roberts intercepted fish that used to feed the Canoe Pass canneries' maw. And so the canning industry slowly declined.

Now, hawks and owls perch on the rotting pilings, taking a temporary respite from their hunts above the marsh and grasslands for Townsend's voles. The land to the east of the dyke trail is farmland that has been temporarily set aside as part of an innovative program between farmers and the Delta Wildlife Trust.

Biologists have planted five different species of grasses to see both how they're used by wildlife and how they improve the soil for agriculture. 'Once we have that information,' says wildlife coordinator Mary Taitt, 'we hope to work out some management strategies.'

Binoculars will help provide a better view of the abundant birdlife that plies the grasslands and the shores surrounding this part of Delta's dyke system, which was built in 1895. In winter, the area hosts an important concentration of trumpeter and tundra swans and snow geese. Among the other species you're likely to see are northern harrier, short-eared owls, killdeer, red-winged blackbirds, marsh wrens and pheasants.

As you mosey farther south, your binoculars will help you espy the two bald eagle nests nestled in a row of windbreak trees. Red-tailed hawks built the first nest, says Taitt, but they were elbowed out by their bigger raptor cousins. The hawks moved a couple of trees down and built another nest, only to be pushed aside again by a second pair of eagles.

As the dyke passes a second farm, the marshlands to the west open to tidal mudflats—the preferred domain of shorebirds, such as sandpipers and sanderlings. It's a great place to watch the constantly shifting clouds of dunlin, palm-sized birds that gather by the hundreds to perform an aerial ballet of light and feather.

From here, there are also clear views—and occasionally sounds—of the trains that run the length of the Roberts Bank jetty to load coal onto foreign freighters. Beyond, just out of sight, is the jetty that runs to the Tsawwassen Ferry Terminal. The occasional blast of a departing ferry can be heard. Beyond that are the distant outlines of the San Juan Islands in the US.

After an easy hour's walk, the dyke passes 34th Street, which is unreachable because of a deep ditch. This spot can be your turnaround point. But if you're still up for more walking, continue further along the dyke to the Roberts Bank jetty. Then retrace your steps to the beginning, this time framed with a distant view of the North Shore mountains.

NORTH VANCOUVER

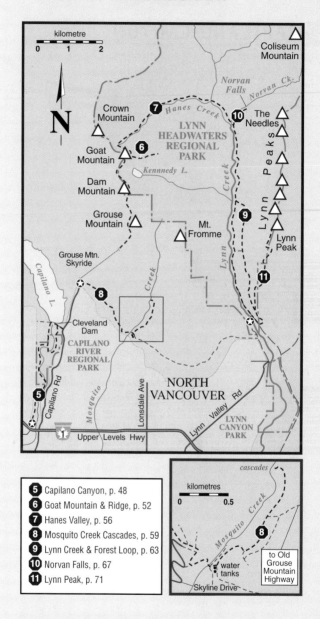

5 Capilano Canyon, p. 48
6 Goat Mountain & Ridge, p. 52
7 Hanes Valley, p. 56
8 Mosquito Creek Cascades, p. 59
9 Lynn Creek & Forest Loop, p. 63
10 Norvan Falls, p. 67
11 Lynn Peak, p. 71

5 CAPILANO CANYON

Distance: 8 km	Rating: Easy
Elevation gain: Minimal	Season: Year-round
High point: 150 m	Topographical map:
Time needed: 2–3 hours	North Vancouver 92G/6
	Trail map: Page 47

Note: Dogs must be leashed.

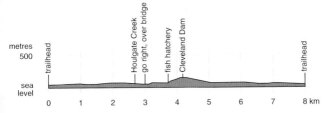

EVEN THE WETTEST WEATHER CAN'T DETER a true hiker for long. So, when raindrops are pelting down and the last place you want to be is in the open, head for the banks of the Capilano River and their thick canopies of hemlock, cedar and fir, which deflect most of the deluge. You'll also find views of the steep-sided granite canyon, remnant big trees and a magnificent manmade waterfall.

To get to the starting point, head for Taylor Way in West Vancouver. About halfway up or downhill, depending on which direction you're coming from, is Keith Road. Turn east (towards North Vancouver) and follow the road past houses and subdivisions over the bridge to where the pavement ends just under the Upper Levels Highway. Park here.

The actual trailhead is just a bit farther along the dirt road, where a yellow gate marks the boundary of the Capilano River Regional Park. Created in 1926, this 160-hectare jewel attracts more than 1 million visitors each year. It is managed by the Greater Vancouver Regional District.

For the first 15 minutes or so, a wide path saunters along the western bank with glimpses of the rushing river down below and the occasional peek at some of the posh homes on the river's steep east bank.

At the first fork in the trail, bear right onto the Capilano Pacific Trail. Just beyond the chain-link fence, you may see the occasional hardy tourist wandering through the forested bits that surround the Capilano Suspension Bridge.

At the second sign, follow a path to the right into the trees, passing through a weathered wooden fence. The real forest trail

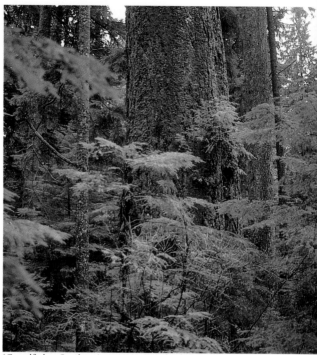

'Grandfather Capilano,' a monster Douglas fir.

is here. Look high to the treetops and feel only a few drops of rain kiss your face. The earlier hum of traffic noise is completely replaced by the rush of the river.

After 10 minutes of walking, the trail forks again. Stay right, closest to the river. Along the way are a couple of viewpoints worth the short detours. One spot has a bench and is the perfect spot for a short water break, while you take in the breathtaking view of canyon and river, named after Chief Kiapalahno, who died in 1870.

Before it was called the Capilano, the river was known to the native residents as Homulcheson Creek. And it was in this part of the river that, legend has it, a chief lived alone in the wilderness for 10 years as a way of protecting his people from the calamities that were supposed to accompany the birth of twins—in this case the chief's own newborn sons. By proving himself stronger than the dark side, the chief could redeem himself and his tribe. And so this chief built a lodge of the firs and cedars, lived off the trout and salmon of the river, the berries and game of the forest and waited for his solitude to end. Pauline Johnson describes the story in the 1911 book.

Legends of Vancouver:

> Then one hot summer day, the Thunderbird came crashing
> through the mountains about him. Up from the arms of the
> Pacific rolled the storm cloud, and the Thunderbird, with its
> eyes of flashing light, beat its huge vibrating wings on crag
> and canyon.... When the beating of those black pinions ceased
> and the echo of their thunder waves died down the depths
> of the canyon, the Squamish Chief arose as a new man. The
> shadow on his soul had lifted, the fears of evil were cowed and
> conquered.

With a new perspective on the river, follow the trail across numerous wooden bridges, some over creeks and streams, and others over tiny bogs. Just after crossing the bridge over Houlgate Creek, the trail forks. Stay right to cross bridge #30, continuing up a small slope to an opening where a number of trails intersect. Turn right to follow the Shinglebolt Trail back to the river. Ten minutes walking brings you out of the trees and on to a gravel path. Go right and over the pipeline bridge.

Here, in Dog Leg Canyon, the river is at its most spectacular. The sharp bend creates whirlpools and boiling, churning waters—the perfect place to contemplate the power of nature.

After crossing the bridge, head left towards Coho Loop and the Capilano River Hatchery. Along the way, you may see folks fishing for steelhead, coho, chinook and chum salmon, which were reared at the hatchery, then released. Operated by the Department of Fisheries and Oceans, the hatchery has excellent educational displays and is open year-round. Call (604) 666–1790 for visiting hours.

Before heading on to Cleveland Dam, take a short stroll to the north end of the parking lot for a look at one of the tallest trees in the Vancouver area. This Douglas fir measures more than 5.5 metres in girth and 76.5 metres in height. Although a few big trees remain, most of the forest giants were logged in the late 1800s and early 1900s. In 1886, a surveyor's report noted that a western red cedar measuring more than 19 metres around was felled.

Then it's on to the Cleveland Dam. The Palisades Trail starts just east of the hatchery, and climbs steepishly for about 500 metres before emerging to a gravel road. Occasionally, deer can be seen grazing on the roadside foliage.

Another 500 metres brings you to the top of the 90-metre-high Cleveland Dam, built in 1954 by the Greater Vancouver Water District and named after Ernest Cleveland, the first Water Commissioner. The pristine waters of Capilano Lake were created when the upper canyon of the river was dammed

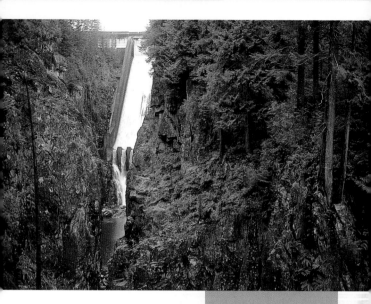

and its valley flooded. Now 80 metres of water covers the trees, squatters' shacks and perhaps a memento or two left behind by early mountaineers. This water is the source of drinking water for the western sector of the Greater Vancouver area.

The views from this manmade precipice are impressive, from the mists that dance around the treetops like water spirits, to the falls that thunder from the lake to the river below.

For the return trip, cross the dam and take the side-trail downhill. Watch for the sign noting the start of the Capilano Pacific Trail and follow it back to the trailhead.

6 GOAT MOUNTAIN AND RIDGE

Distance: 11 km	Rating: Moderate
Elevation gain: 250 m	Season: July to October
High point: 1400 m	Topographical map:
Time needed: 4–5 hours	North Vancouver 92G/6
	Trail map: Page 47

Note: Distance given is from top of the Grouse Mountain Skyride.

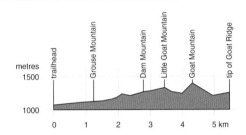

HIKING IS ESSENTIALLY ALL ABOUT getting into the mountains, whether you hike for the views, forests, wildlife, wildflowers, or for just getting away from urban life. Sometimes, though, because of the constraints of time, laziness or physical endurance, you just can't face two or three hours of slogging through rocks, mud and brush-blocked views just to get on top for the good stuff.

Well, here's a hike on which you can cheat. It will, however, cost you the price of a ticket on the Grouse Mountain Skyride—the instant gratification gateway to a number of peaks contained within the backcountry of Lynn Headwaters Regional Park.

Our objective is Goat Mountain and its nearby ridge. En route, there are few steep sections, except for the scramble to the top. Still, the footing can be tricky in places thanks to tangles of tree roots and some loose rock.

To get to the trailhead, head for Capilano Road just east of the dividing line between West Vancouver and North Vancouver. Follow Capilano Road north, past Cleveland Dam where the road becomes Nancy Greene Way, right to the very end. Park in the Grouse lot.

Take the Skyride up, enjoying the grunt-free views of Vancouver, Capilano Lake and the Strait of Georgia. Once at the top, follow the paved path towards the peak chair. About 500 metres along, a wide dirt road sweeps around the west slope of Grouse Mountain proper. The mountain received its

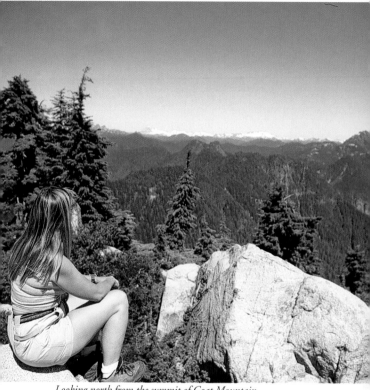

Looking north from the summit of Goat Mountain.

name when, in 1894, a blue grouse found itself in the wrong place at the wrong time, and was shot by the first party to climb the peak.

Fifteen to 20 minutes of walking brings you to the trailhead proper, conveniently located next to a hiker registration board. Sign in—from here on you enter wilderness and all the uncertainties that come with it.

Pass through the wooden gate and head up the trail. Ten to 15 minutes later are signposts indicating the way to Dam, Goat and Crown mountains. We'll stay on the trail straight ahead, towards Goat. This mountain, too, takes its name from two unlucky animals who were shot, also in 1894, by the first party that climbed this peak; this time the animals were mountain goats. (Whether it was the same folks who bagged the grouse is not recorded.)

Another 15 to 20 minutes of walking brings you to Little Goat. Here, from a perfectly placed wilderness bench, is the first view of Goat Mountain and Ridge, with Coliseum Mountain off in the distance. Stop for a water break or a dawdle, and visit with the gray jays who will want to make your acquaintance, especially if you have any food.

The ascent of Little Goat and the other peaks here wasn't always this easy. Before the days of ski lifts and skyrides, before the Capilano watershed was closed to the public, access to Grouse, Dam and Goat—as well as Mount Strachan and The Lions—was made via the Capilano Valley.

As you continue along the trail through open forest, look way down (on the right) below the trail for a peek of Kennedy Lake—once known as the 'Pearl of the Mountains'—part of Greater Vancouver's water supply. Soon come more signposts. Follow the trail to the right.

Where the trail splits next, go right again towards Goat and Crown mountains. An interesting historical note on Crown is that, in 1904, North Vancouver pioneer Charles Mee had big plans to build a resort on its 1500-metre summit. In addition to a chalet and central restaurant, Mee envisioned several cottages available for lease by the day or week. But the resort was never built, nor was the railway once planned to the top of Grouse.

Another 10 to 15 minutes on the trail brings you to the first prominence of Goat Ridge. If you're new to hiking and have had enough, this spot can be the turnaround point for a two- to three-hour return hike.

If not, push on through a steepish section of trail. At one point—about 15 to 20 minutes in—a braided rope is there to help pull yourself up a particularly vertical chunk of the path. Then bear right and follow the orange markers. Another 10 to 15 minutes brings you to a signpost and a point of decision.

Which to do first, Goat Mountain (left) or Goat Ridge (right)? Go right and have lunch away from the crowds that often gather on the summit. Save the 45-minute side-trip ascent of Mount Goat for the return. A five-minute ramble along the ridge should find a picnic spot without much company except the stunning 360° views. To the east are Lynn Peak and Coliseum Mountain; behind them Mount Seymour, Mount Elsay and stately Cathedral Mountain are clearly visible to the northeast. Farther beyond are mountains, mountains, mountains, as far as the eye can see.

To the north is Sky Pilot, the highest of the summits east of the head of Howe Sound. To the southeast are glimpses of Mount Baker and Indian Arm. To the southwest are views of the Lower Mainland, the Strait of Georgia and Vancouver Island in the distance.

If you've read Pauline Johnson's *Legends of Vancouver*, you may feel a chill of recognition. In the story titled 'The Lost Island,' a great medicine man climbs through 'mighty forests' and 'trailless deep mosses and matted vines' to the summit of Grouse Mountain. There, after many days of camping, fasting and singing medicine songs, he is given the power to see far into the future.

> He looked across a hundred years, just as he looked across what you call the Inlet, and he saw mighty lodges built close together, hundreds and thousands of them; lodges built of stone and wood, and long, straight trails to divide them.
>
> He saw these trails thronging with Palefaces; he heard the sound of the white man's paddle-dip on the waters, for it is not silent like the Indian's; he saw the white man's trading posts, saw the fishing nets, heard his speech.

Once you're ready to depart, retrace your steps to civilization and the Skyride.

7 HANES VALLEY

Distance: 17 km

Elevation gain: Minimal

High point: 1425 m

Time needed: 6–7 hours

Rating: Challenging

Season: Late July to September

Topographical map:
North Vancouver 92G/6

Trail map: Page 47

Note: Arrange transportation from Lynn Headwaters back to Grouse. Call BC Transit at (604) 521–0400 for bus schedule information.

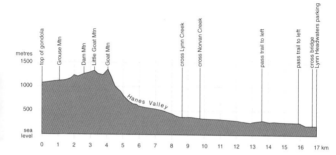

NOT ALL HIKING CHALLENGES ARE IN THE realm of the physical. Sometimes you need more brain than brawn, more sense than stamina to get you safely from point A to B and home again.

The trail to Hanes Valley is within the boundaries of Lynn Headwaters Regional Park and is, for the most part, well-marked. But there are sections, such as a kilometre-long boulder field, where finding one's way is not an easy task. As well, 17 kilometres over rough terrain makes for a long day, even for veteran hikers.

To get to the trailhead, head for Capilano Road just east of the dividing line between West Vancouver and North Vancouver. Follow Capilano Road north, past Cleveland Dam where the road becomes Nancy Greene Way, right to the very end. Park in the Grouse lot.

Now, on to the trail. The starting point is the top of Grouse Mountain. It's best to take the Skyride to the

> Despite the mild elevation statistics, this hike is not for beginners or, for that matter, many intermediate hikers. Hanes Valley is best left until you have acquired the ability to use a map and compass (I do mean **use** them, not just carry them).

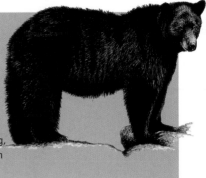

In late summer, blueberry bushes line the trail, with plump and juicy fruit. Remember though, where there are berries, there will likely be bears. So make noise—talk, sing, whistle—to alert them to your presence.

top, but if you're a purist—or a glutton for punishment—you could spend 90 minutes to two hours slogging up the Grouse Grind Trail.

Once off the Skyride, follow the concrete towards the Peak Chair, which you will not take. Instead follow a wide dirt road, which curls around the west side of Grouse's true peak. Within 20 minutes of leaving Grouse is the park sign-in board. Fill out one of the registration slips. Be sure to sign in.

Now, head up the trail. After 10 to 15 minutes are signposts indicating trails to Dam, Goat and Crown mountains. Take the trail straight ahead. Another 15 to 20 minutes brings you to Little Goat, with views of Goat Mountain and Ridge, and Coliseum Mountain in the distance.

The trail then scoots through open forest, which, if you look down on the right, allows a peek of Kennedy Lake, part of Greater Vancouver's water supply. Soon after, the trail splits. Folks heading for Goat Mountain continue straight ahead. But we will bear left, towards Crown Pass and beyond to Hanes Valley. Just a few steps brings you to a bluff with views of Crown Mountain and the double-humped Camel Mountain. Soak up the high altitude views, because it's all downhill from here.

Even though you're descending, the trail is not easy. Rather, it is damnably steep with muddy sections that require some fancy footwork and wet rocky sections where you must pay attention. Be thankful you're not grunting up the same slope, and take your time working your way down.

After 30 to 40 minutes of descent, the trail reaches Crown Pass and the intersection with the Crown Mountain Trail. Continue straight ahead—stopping at the eastern lip of the pass for the first view of Hanes Valley. In late summer, the valley looks like a wilderness crib, with steep rock walls and a green blanket of berry bush.

Continue the descent to the beginning of a vast boulder

field—your best stop for a lunch break (it's relatively bug-free, has great views and immediately precedes an hour or so of painstakingly picking your way among wobbly rocks).

After lunch, you will need those finely honed route-finding skills. Although some orange flags can be seen fluttering in the boulder field, others have been laid low by snow, falling rock and other mountain elements. You must stay on track to pick up the trail lower down where it enters the forest. If you get off track, you could find yourself lost in the big beyond. Once again, if you don't have the necessary route-finding skills, save the hike for a later time or go with a grizzled hiking veteran.

After an hour of picking through the boulder field, the trail enters the forest—a welcome respite of green, especially if the day is hot and the boulder field is like a furnace. Soon, you'll hear the tinkle of Hanes Creek.

The creek gets its name from George Hanes, who was the engineer for North Vancouver in the 1920s and '30s. Together with Reeve Julius Fromme (after whom Fromme Mountain is named), Hanes regularly travelled the wilderness of the Lynn Creek Watershed to make inspections and note needed improvements.

Soon, the trail comes to a signpost that marks the halfway point between Grouse and Lynn Headwaters. Have a blueberry in celebration, take in the views up the Hanes Valley—as magnificent as they were from the top. And continue on, traversing through the forest along a real trail with real markers again (yahoo!). The path crosses a few tributaries of Hanes Creek and about an hour later reaches Lynn Creek. Here, the waters seems to spill from pool to pool, each a cool temptation. Leave yourself enough time to indulge in at least a foot-dunking.

When you're ready, follow the yellow markers and trail into the forest. Along the way are remnants of Lynn Valley's logging days: big stumps with springboard holes, the occasional rusting cable and other artifacts—porcelain shards, rusted stove parts, glittering pieces of broken bottle. Look, touch, but don't take anything with you.

After 30 minutes, you'll come to Norvan Creek and, most likely, run into other hikers who've made the Norvan Falls their day-trip destination. Another 45 minutes of walking along a wide corduroy road will bring you to a debris chute and more people. Stay along the creek for an easy hike to the Lynn Headwaters Regional Park parking lot. Or head left and into the trees for a quieter, but steeper, ending. Be sure to deposit your registration stub in the box on the signboard before crossing the Lynn Creek bridge.

MOSQUITO CREEK CASCADES 8

Distance: 8 km	Rating: Moderate
Elevation gain: 320 m	Season: March to November
High point: 600 m	Topographical map:
Time needed: Up to 5 hours	North Vancouver 92G/6
	Trail map: Page 47

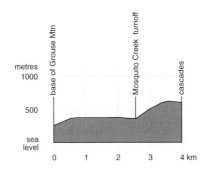

MANY A HIKER FIRST SETS FOOT ON THE trails of the North Shore mountains. These days, it seems, more and more people are discovering the delights of getting out in the great outdoors. Still, there are trails that are rarely trodden, sights less often seen. This outing reveals one of those better-kept secrets—the Mosquito Creek Cascades.

Although it is possible to start from various access points along the way, we'll start from the parking lot at Grouse Mountain and incorporate a scenic portion of the Baden-Powell Trail for a well-rounded day.

Drive to Capilano Road, just east of the dividing line between West Vancouver and North Vancouver. Follow Capilano Road north, past Cleveland Dam where the road becomes Nancy Greene Way, and keep going right to the very end. Park in the Grouse lot.

From the lot, head east to find the start of the trail. Almost immediately, the way heads up along a well-worn trail. Five minutes later, you'll come to the turnoff point for the Grouse Grind Trail—the reason for all the wear and tear. While hundreds of hikers head off for one of the least-scenic, least-rewarding but most-hyped trails on the North Shore, you continue straight ahead.

The trail grinds steadily upward through second-growth forest with a rich understorey of ferns, huckleberry bush and

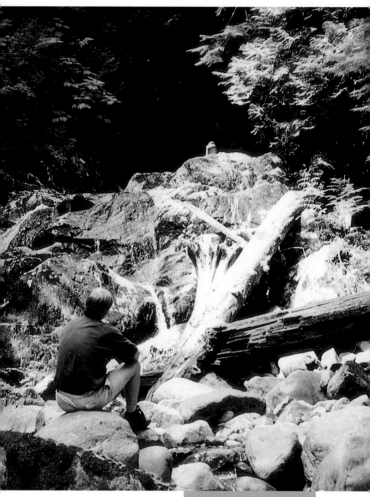

mosses. After 30 to 40 minutes the trail levels off and passes its first junction with the old BC Mountaineering Club (BCMC) trail. Continue straight to cross the first tributary of MacKay Creek.

In summer, the Mosquito Creek Cascades are a cool idyll to take respite from the heat of the day and the bustle of the city.

Then, 10 minutes later, is the main channel for MacKay.

During 1996's big fall rains, MacKay became a torrent of water, flooding houses farther downslope and carving the creekbed right down to bedrock. Downed trees still litter the waterway. And you can see where the torrent also washed out the trail. Take care when scrambling down and up the steepish sides to cross the creek.

Another 10 minutes brings you to the second junction with the old BCMC trail. Fifteen minutes later, civilization intrudes on the forest, first as suburban noise, then as old paved roads and new houses.

At a major junction, signs point left to a trail that follows the old Grouse Mountain chairlift, and right to the continuing Baden-Powell. Go right and follow the sign pointing toward Skyline Drive. But instead of descending all the way, go only about 25 metres before taking the trail east towards Mosquito Creek.

A wooden bridge once crossed the creek, but in the fall of 1996 it was washed out by floodwaters. You'll have to boulder hop across the creek—carefully—to the next leg of your explorations. Follow the trail towards the two big water towers. Just behind them, along the creek's east side, a small trail veers off for a short easy stroll to see the remnants of an old dam.

Once back on the main trail, continue only about 10 metres past the water towers. Look on the left for markers indicating 'Old Grouse Mountain Highway, 50 min.' and follow the trail up.

The trail is built along the remnants of a pipeline that once fed drinking water from Kennedy Lake to the city of North Vancouver. In the early 1980s, a storm destroyed the intake and it was decided that the cost of restoring the system couldn't be justified. Pieces of the pipe are still visible, and there's even the occasional rusting fire plug that bears the name 'Terminal City Ironworks.'

After 15 minutes of a steep ascent, you'll see a big Douglas fir, its lower trunk scarred black by a fire that swept the North Shore in the 1930s. Remnants of an old cabin can also be seen.

The trail then zigs away from the creek and into the forest. You're walking on one of a maze of skid roads in the area which can make it easy to get confused, so pay close attention to the markers here. On the left of the trail, watch for a big rock and the markers just on the far side, which note an important turn. Go left here.

Fifteen minutes of gradual uphill walking brings you to a trail junction. Right goes to the old Grouse Mountain Highway, but we'll go straight to follow the signs that note the viewpoint and cascades not far ahead. This part of the trail doesn't see many visitors, so there'll be places where you'll have to climb over recent deadfall and detour around big downed trees and slimy rocky bits laid bare by slumps.

In about 15 minutes is a point with views of Lions Gate Bridge, the west side of Vancouver and farther out to sea. The next few minutes take you through a section of the forest dotted with big stumps and springboard holes that look like eyes.

In the 1910s, a small shingle mill was built on Mosquito Creek to process trees cut on the slopes of Grouse just above the creek. A few small summer cottages once perched in the area and a log bridge once spanned the creek. However, more massive logging operations upslope caused drastic changes in a short period of time, as John Davidson, the first provincial botanist and first president of the Vancouver Natural History Society noted in a 1924 address:

> Within two years a large scar made its appearance. Trees, gravel and rocks were washed down; at least one of the houses was smashed by falling trees; debris temporarily dammed the creek, washed out the bridge and its supports of rock, and deposited sand, gravel, rocks and trees all along the lower part of the valley. Spring freshets are now an annual menace, the erosion continues, the end is not yet. The scar can now be seen from Vancouver and is increasing year by year. Other scars are beginning, and will soon be in evidence from this side.

For Davidson, the damage caused by such massive deforestation as took place on the North Shore in the 1920s was the 'writing on the wall.' An investigation was sparked by Davidson and others, and logging was halted in the Capilano watershed.

Fortunately, some of the big trees of Mosquito Creek are still in place along the trail—Douglas fir at first, then western red cedar lower down. Follow the trail carefully to the rocky banks of Mosquito Creek. In spring, the water rushes through in one long whitewater torrent.

After a long lunch break, return to the Baden-Powell Trail, cross Mosquito Creek and continue until you see the orange-roofed house below. Then, go straight instead of following the Baden-Powell upwards. Follow the paved road on which you'll emerge to the power line and the gravel road that runs beneath it. It's an easy 20 to 25 minutes back to the parking lot amid open skies and urban wildflowers.

LYNN CREEK & FOREST LOOP 9

Distance: 9.5 km	Season: Year-round
Elevation gain: Minimal	Topographical map:
High point: 350 m	North Vancouver 92G/6
Time needed: 3–4 hours	Trail map: Page 47
Rating: Easy	Note: Dogs must be leashed.

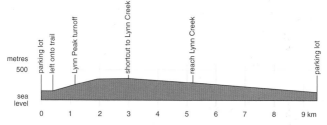

O NE OF THE GREAT THINGS ABOUT LYNN Headwaters Regional Park is a loop system that allows for a tremendous variety of trip lengths—from a short jaunt of two hours to a longish trek of five to six hours. The park is a perfect year-round destination, negotiable in just about any weather.

To get to the trailhead, take the Lynn Canyon exit off the Upper Levels Highway and follow Lynn Valley Road north, past the turnoff to Lynn Canyon Park, to the very end. The green and yellow GVRD signs then lead to the parking areas.

Cross the bridge over Lynn Creek to the signboard with hiker registration. After filling in a slip, go right and up an old gravel road to the yellow metal gate that marks the boundary between Lynn Headwaters and the Lower Seymour Conservation Reserve. Go left to follow the Lynn Loop Trail.

After a short uphill section, the trail levels and wanders through a mossy green cathedral of western red cedar, western hemlock and the occasional Douglas fir and Sitka spruce.

A few big trees still remain, but the huge stumps of their now-fallen relatives are more impressive. The stumps date back about a century, when, after having cut most of the North Shore in the 1890s, loggers turned their attention to the big trees of Lynn Valley.

Some trees, including the biggest Douglas fir ever taken from Lynn Valley, took three days to fell. This forest giant was recorded as being more than 13 metres in circumference;

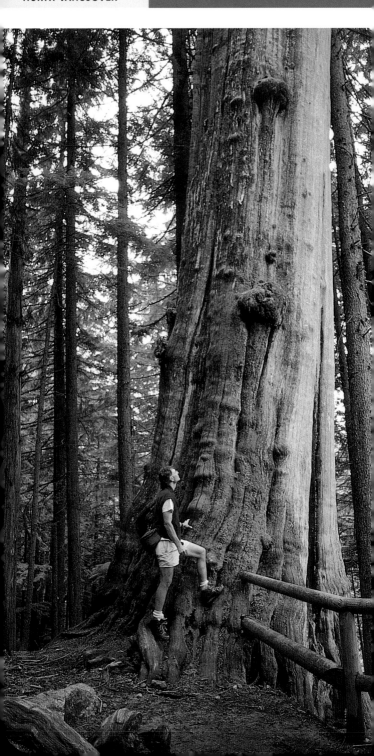

the bark alone was 36 centimetres thick. The height of the tree was estimated at more than 120 metres, making it more than 20 metres taller than the Marine Building in downtown Vancouver.

Imagine walking through an entire forest of such giants as you continue past the side-trail on the right leading to Lynn Peak. About 3 kilometres in, a trail on the left drops to Lynn Creek for a short two-hour loop. We, however, will continue straight ahead, soaking up the sights and smells of West Coast rainforest.

Eventually, the trail emerges to a clearing known as the Second Debris Chute. This spot is the point of second return along the creek. Although the trail continues farther north to Norvan Falls, Hanes Valley and Lynn Lake, we'll make this our turnaround point.

Head west towards the sound of the creek. Before it was given its present name, this creek was called Kwalcha by the Squamish people who lived on its banks. In 1863, after the first non-Natives settled, its name was recorded as Fred's Creek, after pre-emptor Frederick Howson. But in later years, it was named Lynn after John Linn. (Unfortunately, the record didn't quite spell the name correctly.)

Linn, one of a contingent of Royal Engineers, came to BC in 1859. When the unit disbanded four years later, he settled with his family at the mouth of Lynn Creek. Linn's barnyard menagerie included horses, cows and poultry, but he didn't raise pigs, because pigs were often carried off by resident cougars.

The path along the river is called the Cedars Mill Trail. In 1917, the Cedars Ltd. Sawmill was built on the east bank of Lynn Creek. Although a logging railway had been planned for the upper valley, trucks—the first to be used in the province—were instead used to haul felled trees. A plank road about a car-lane wide was built to Norvan Creek.

Work crews, made up mainly of Swedish and Japanese immigrants, worked the upper valley. Their camps became known as Shaketown because of the production of cedar shakes and shingles there. Remains of the camps can still be found—pieces of rusted machinery, an occasional old boot or shattered tea cup. Fires raged through the area in 1910 and 1920. In 1925, fire struck again, killing a worker. Three years later, the area was designated for water supply and the old Cedars Mill was closed.

Depending on which time of year you hike along the eastern bank, Lynn Creek can be either a burbling stream or

Western red cedar, Lynn Forest.

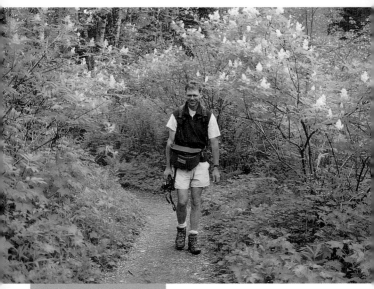

The trails lead through all sorts of beautiful terrain—fragrant groves of alder and aspen, cedar-spired forest cathedrals, dense skunky scented marsh and, of course, the clear, rushing waters of Lynn Creek.

a rushing torrent. The creek begins high in the mountains as snow and ice. From its melt-water beginnings, it is joined by other feeder creeks on the way downstream, eventually spilling into Burrard Inlet, 20 kilometres distant.

Its clean, clear beginnings made Lynn a perfect candidate for fresh drinking water. From 1928 to 1985 the Upper Lynn watershed was closed to the public. But a 1981 storm washed out the water intakes, altered the course of the creek and destroyed part of the east side road. Replacement was judged to be too expensive, so Greater Vancouver got a big, beautiful new wilderness park.

As you cross the pebbles and stones that mark the old wash-out and head back along a wide, tree-canopied road, look just off the trail for remnants of the old intake pipe—wooden staves and steel rings. Before you know it, you'll be back to the signboard where you can deposit the remaining half of your sign-in slip and head home.

NORVAN FALLS 10

Distance: 13.5 km	Rating: Moderate
Elevation gain: Minimal	Season: Year-round
High point: 375 m	Topographical map:
Time needed: 5–6 hours	North Vancouver 92G/6
	Trail map: Page 47

Note: Dogs must be leashed.

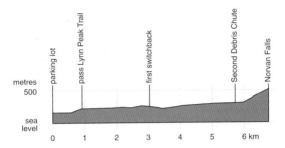

I N WINTER OR SPRING, A SHORT WALK IN THE woods sometimes just can't satisfy your hiking desires. With snow still on the mountains, alpine outings are still weeks or months away.

But there's a place for a hiker to go for a good trail-pounding fix, both long enough to feel like a real hike, but moderate enough to be gentle on unacclimatized leg muscles. Norvan Falls is a great spring or winter destination, especially when there's just enough snow and frost to make it a winter wonderland.

To get to the trailhead, follow the Upper Levels Highway to North Vancouver and take the Lynn Canyon exit. Follow Lynn Valley Road north to the very end. (Don't take the turn to Lynn Canyon Park; keep going straight.) Then watch for the green and yellow GVRD signs to point you to the parking area and the trailhead proper.

Cross the bridge over Lynn Creek to the park signboard and sign in at the hiker registration. To get the most out of the hike to Norvan Falls, head right on a wide road towards the yellow gate that marks the boundary between Lynn Headwaters and the Lower Seymour Conservation Reserve. Just on the left is the start of the Lynn Loop Trail. After a short uphill section, the trail levels and meanders through sweetly scented groves of western red cedar, western hemlock and the occasional Douglas fir or Sitka spruce.

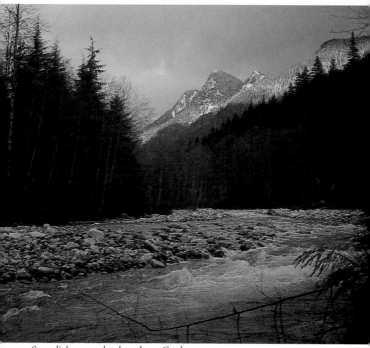

Stormlight on peaks above Lynn Creek.

Most of the trees are second-growth, their predecessors having been reduced to stumps by logging. In the early 1900s, trees here grew as high as some of modern Vancouver's tallest office buildings. Imagine what it would have been like to wander through such a grove.

Soon is the junction with the trail to Lynn Peak. About 3 kilometres later, on the left, are the switchbacks that drop to Lynn Creek. Continue straight, absorbing all the nuances of the West Coast rainforest for another couple of kilometres.

Eventually, the trail emerges to a clearing known as the Second Debris Chute. While it's possible to double back and return along the creek, we'll keep heading northward. If there is snow and ice on the first part of the trail, you will want to carefully consider where your feet are planted, so you don't inadvertently go 'tobogganing.'

The remaining 3 kilometres of trail to Norvan Creek are even more peaceful than those you've travelled thus far. Fewer people ply these footways than the earlier parts of the trail. A good portion of the trail still shows the corduroy road put down by loggers earlier in the 20th century.

Before the arrival of non-Natives, the forest was untouched except for the occasional cedar that was felled to make a dug-out canoe. However, notes North Vancouver pioneer Walter Draycott in his book *Early Days in Lynn Valley*, 'when the white man gazed in amazement upon the magnificent forest, his first thought was of masts for sailing ships.' Soon the 'white man' had a few more thoughts, and trees were felled as building material for houses, boardwalks, furniture and a hundred other things.

The 25-metre cascade tumbles down rock, which is actually the edge of a big mass of granite that, millions of years ago, pushed its way into older rock below the Earth's surface. The surrounding older rock was affected by all the heat and pressure to produce copper, lead and zinc sulphides that would become of particular interest to miners.

The Lynn Valley Lumber Company is cited by Draycott as providing 'first-class fir and cedar.' At the time, western hemlock had little value, except, as Draycott notes, 'with the squirrels and owls.'

In 1925, the last stand of virgin Douglas firs was felled in the district of North Vancouver. 'They had attained a height of 150 to 250 feet with diameters ranging from 4 to 9 feet, excluding bark,' writes Draycott of the fallen giants. 'The bark on the larger trees was 12 to 14 inches thick.' The stand was turned into 1 million board feet of commercial timber, with one particularly fine fir responsible for 30,000 board feet alone.

As well, notes Draycott, 'on the upper branches of the tallest giants were several eagles' nests—which may account for the reluctance of the Indians to have the trees destroyed.'

Suddenly, the forest looks a little different, perhaps a little lonely. Eventually, the old corduroy road ends at Norvan Creek—although there once were plans to extend the road to Lynn Lake. Where the trail forks go right and upstream for a short walk to the falls.

The area was, in fact, home to mining activity in the early 1900s. The old Mountain Lion and Copper Duke claims explored zinc and copper deposits just south of Norvan Creek. The trails leading to the claims are long overgrown. But some remnant tunnels, shafts and cuts lie just below the forest floor, so it's best not to go off-trail.

After a lunch break and a viewing of the falls, it's time to hit the trail again. Simply retrace your steps to the Second Debris Chute. Instead of following the same route that brought you here, take in the creekside scenery along the Cedars Mill Trail.

It's different terrain and foliage than you've seen thus far—open glades of bare-branched alder and birch, the new green leaves of huckleberry bush and, of course, the icy tumble of Lynn Creek. When you reach the signboard, remember to deposit the other half of your registration slip.

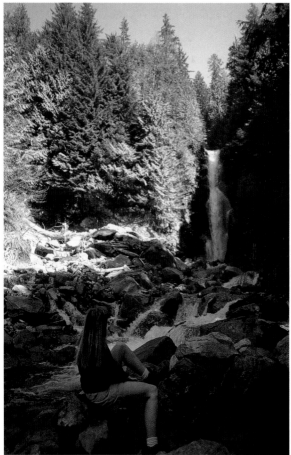

Norvan Falls is the reward at the end of the trail.

LYNN PEAK

11

Distance: 7 km

Elevation gain: 700 m

High point: 920 m

Time needed: 4 hours

Rating: Moderate

Season: May to November

Topographical map:
North Vancouver 92G/6

Trail map: Page 47

Note: Dogs must be leashed.

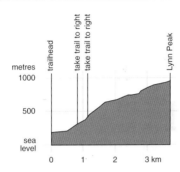

N OT MANY PEOPLE SEEM TO HAVE BEEN TO Lynn Peak, and few people seem to have any interest in seeking it out. But it's a day-trip well worth making for its old-growth trees, terrific views and geological walk through time. It's also close enough to the city that you won't need to get up at 6 a.m. just to ensure finishing during daylight hours.

To get to the trailhead, take the Lynn Canyon exit in North Vancouver off the Upper Levels Highway. Follow Lynn Valley Road past the turnoff to Lynn Canyon Park, right to the road's end. Then follow the green-and-yellow GVRD signs to the parking area and trailhead proper at Lynn Headwaters Regional Park.

Cross the bridge and sign in at the hiker registration. Part of the registration slip goes in now; the other part when you return safe and sound. Take note of any advisories, such as the presence of bears or cougars. Then follow the wide gravel road to the right and to the yellow metal gate that marks the boundary between Lynn Headwaters and the Lower Seymour Conservation Reserve. Go left to follow the Lynn Loop Trail.

The trail wanders among western red cedar, western hemlock and the occasional Douglas fir or Sitka spruce. A few big trees still remain, but it's the stumps that are most impressive. Before loggers turned their attention to the big trees of Lynn Valley in the early 1900s, many trees grew as tall as downtown

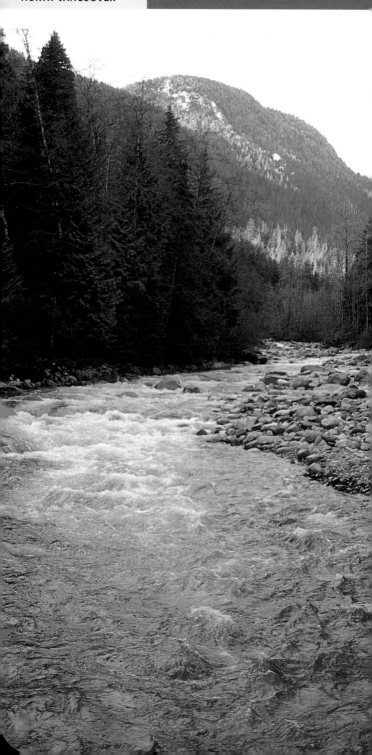

office buildings. The biggest Douglas fir felled in Lynn Valley measured more than 120 metres high—20 metres taller than the art deco Marine Building in downtown Vancouver.

> From the 920-metre summit, there are gorgeous views of Burrard Inlet, Seymour Demonstration Forest and Rice Lake, the peaks of Seymour Mountain and on and on.

Soon, the trail to Lynn Peak bears right from the main path. Look for the sign right beside the Three Sisters—a troika of big burned-out stumps. From here on, follow the square yellow trail markers—and occasional orange tape—attached to tree trunks and branches.

For the first hour or so, the trail heads up steeply and steadily. Take a water break every 15 minutes or so and contemplate the ground you're walking on. Or rather, the rock beneath it—quartz diorite, the same 85-million- to 140-million-year-old rock that makes up most of the North Shore mountains. It's different from the relatively young sediments of sand, silt, clay and gravel surrounding Lynn Creek that were laid down within the last 8000 or so years.

The trail eventually reaches the first viewpoint with somewhat closed-in views of Seymour Mountain. Far below, the Seymour River rumbles.

From here, the trail heads into a lovely grove of old-growth spruce, fir and cedar known as 'The Enchanted Forest.' There's a palpable hush in the air, except for the occasional *rat-a-tat-tat* of a woodpecker looking for lunch in a snag. At times, you may feel that if you just turn that next corner, you'll find some old crone with an enticing gingerbread house.

About 30 to 40 minutes later—cookie fantasies aside—is a second viewpoint, just off-trail past a few small trees. From here there are more open views of Seymour and all its peaks. You can now see as well as hear the Seymour River below.

This spot is known as the Blimp Lookout, after the Zeppelin-type dirigible that was moored here in the 1960s as part of a balloon logging operation attempting to salvage trees downed in 1962's Hurricane Frieda. The slopes were considered too steep for more traditional retrieval methods. But before all the big trees were hauled out, the blimp was destroyed in a 1967 storm.

After a water break, push on again. Another 20 to 25 minutes later is yet another viewpoint, this one looking out to Greater Vancouver as it stretches off towards the US border and into

Lynn Creek near trailhead.

the Fraser Valley. On a clear day, you can see Vancouver Island and some of the San Juan and Gulf islands.

As you continue on, the rock under the ground under your feet has changed yet again. This time, it's gabbro, a coarse dark rock. In all likelihood, the gabbro was here first, then the quartz diorite described earlier was forced in as magma, under the Earth's surface.

Digest that info as you continue for another 15 to 20 minutes to the sign pointing to your final destination—Lynn Peak. You're literally on top of the final geological oddity of the day: metamorphosed volcanic rocks. They're part of what's known as the Gambier Group, a layer of older volcanic and sedimentary rock that was partly absorbed by the magma that oozed its way to the top.

Once you've had a good look around, a rest and some lunch, retrace your steps to the signboard at Lynn Creek. Don't forget to put the registration slip in the box before you cross the footbridge.

NORTH VANCOUVER

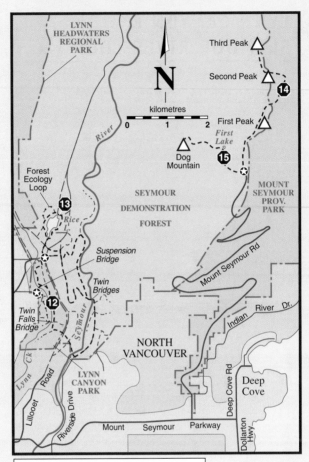

LYNN HEADWATERS REGIONAL PARK

Third Peak

Second Peak

14

kilometres

0   1   2

First Peak

First Lake

Dog Mountain

15

Forest Ecology Loop

13

Rice L.

MOUNT SEYMOUR PROV. PARK

SEYMOUR

DEMONSTRATION

FOREST

Suspension Bridge

Twin Bridges

Mount Seymour Rd

12

Twin Falls Bridge

Seymour

Lynn Ck

Indian   River   Dr.

NORTH VANCOUVER

LYNN CANYON PARK

Deep Cove Rd

Deep Cove

Lillooet   Road

Riverside Drive

Dollarton Hwy

Mount   Seymour   Parkway

---

12 Lynn Canyon & Seymour River Loop, p. 76

13 Seymour River & Rice Lake Loop, p. 81

14 Mount Seymour, p. 85

15 Dog Mountain, p. 88

12 LYNN CANYON & SEYMOUR RIVER LOOP

Distance: Up to 8 km

Elevation gain: Minimal

High point: 320 m

Time needed: Up to 3 hours

Rating: Easy

Season: Year-round

Topographical map:
North Vancouver 92G/6

Trail map: Page 75

Note: Dogs are not allowed in Seymour Demonstration Forest.

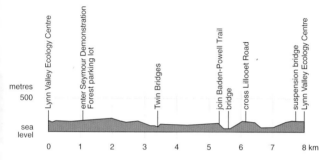

IN WINTER, WHEN YOU DON'T HAVE THE luxury of long, warm sunny days, you want options in your outings, just in case the drizzle turns to downpour or you underestimate the hours of available light.

The hike to Lynn Canyon and the Seymour River Loop spans parts of two North Shore parks—Lynn Canyon and the Lower Seymour Conservation Reserve—and is full of choices. A shorter route takes about 90 minutes; a longer outing about three hours.

The starting point for both routes is Lynn Canyon Park. To get there, take the Lynn Valley Road exit off the Upper Levels Highway and head north. Follow the signs to Lynn Canyon (not Lynn Headwaters) Park and find a spot in the lot. The park, created in 1912, is the oldest in the municipality of North Vancouver.

First stop is the Lynn Canyon suspension bridge, with its views of Lynn Creek churning 80 metres below. The original suspension bridge, built in 1912, was a commercial venture with owner and district councillor J.P. Crawford charging a 10-cent toll to people who wished to cross. In later years, the bridge became decrepit and was closed. Not long after, the

Lynn Creek, below suspension bridge.

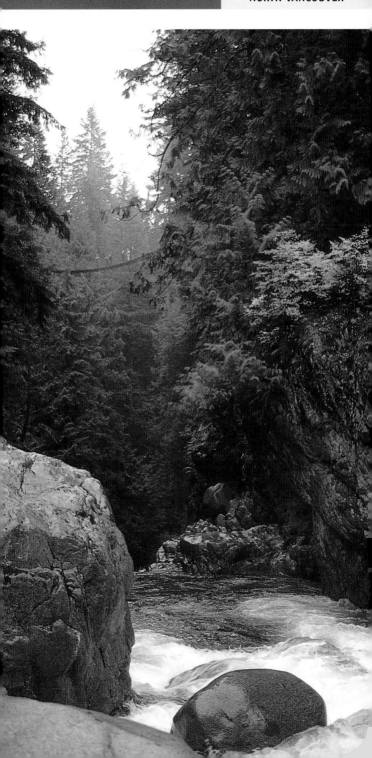

> The trail winds down, down, down through second-growth forest to the Seymour River through a lush green forest of western hemlock, western red cedar and moss-covered vine maple and alder.

district of North Vancouver took it over, repaired and renovated the classic span and removed the fee.

Few people walk farther than the other side of the bridge. We, however, will head up a short flight of wooden stairs on the left and continue to follow the trail as it bears left. The trail winds alongside Lynn Creek through often muddy, wet and slippery ground. Soon, the trail leads to the foot of a long set of wooden stairs. About 100 metres beyond the top of the stairs, the trail forks. Go left along the flat ground through open forest.

Another seven minutes brings you to the path and bridge that connect Lynn Headwaters Regional Park and the Lower Seymour Conservation Reserve, both administered by the Greater Vancouver Regional District. Head right (east) along the gravel path, which leads to the SDF's parking lot. Continue straight across, following the path into the trees. At the yellow gate, go right. About 100 metres farther, go left on the Homestead Trail. (Right leads to Twin Bridges.)

The Homestead Trail meets with the Fisherman's Trail as it winds along the Seymour River. Go right, walking along what used to be a road, through copses of alder, maple and cottonwood. On the left, notice the now-mossy gate of a former homestead, and, a little farther, the moss-covered arches of another.

Before the Seymour Valley was designated a watershed in the 1920s, a small community existed along the river's edge. You can still see old fenceposts, gates, chimneys and foundations, remnants of the homes and ranches that once were here.

The trail meanders along the river. In about 20 minutes, you'll come across another artifact from the past—a tunnel cut into the rock. A wooden water pipeline once ran through here. The pipe, completed in 1907, carried clean, clear Seymour River water beneath the Second Narrows to the City of Vancouver.

(Lower on the Seymour River, some shafts were also cut into rock by would-be gold miners in the mid- to late 1800s. Some gold was found, but never enough to warrant a full-fledged mine.)

A few minutes later, the trail comes to an intersection at Twin Bridges. Here, you face a decision. If you want to make

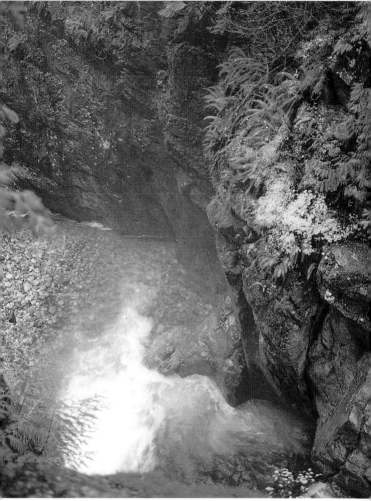

Lynn Creek, Lynn Canyon.

this spot the turnaround point for a short 5-kilometre round trip, follow the trail right and uphill back to the parking lot, then retrace your steps to Lynn Canyon.

Otherwise, continue on the longer jaunt, over the intact twin of the Twin Bridges and onto the trail on the east side of Seymour River. After 10 to 15 minutes of walking, the trail forks. Continue straight and cross the wooden bridge with log rails. Another 10 minutes brings you to another fork in the trail. Here, go left and up a slight incline. (Right is the old trail, now washed out and impassable.)

Not much farther is sudden civilization, in the form of houses on a cul-de-sac. Just before the wooden-railed pipe bridge that would lead you further into the subdivision, look for a trail to the right, which leads down to another pipe bridge lined with chain-link fencing.

Now, you're on part of the Baden-Powell Trail. Cross the bridge and ooh over the spectacular sight of the Seymour River as it thunders through a narrow gorge. Now comes a flight of stairs. After 55 steep steps, follow the trail (with its square orange markers) as it bears left.

The sound of the river recedes as the trail continue its upward slog. Soon, you enter the quiet of the forest. After 10 to 20 minutes of uphill, the trail crosses a concrete pipeline and emerges under a power line. The snow-capped peaks of Mount Seymour are visible in the distance.

At an intersection, continue straight for a few minutes of easy walking to the gravel of Lillooet Road. Cross it, then bear left for about 50 metres to pick up the continuation of the Baden-Powell Trail.

As the trail heads into the forest, the sounds of Lynn Creek seep through the trees, as well as the occasional view of distant peaks. A few minutes later, the trail comes to a signpost and map. Follow the trail directly downhill until you finally reach a boardwalk over marshy ground to the creek's edge. The trail meanders along the mist-draped creek through some muddy, wet and slippery sections, so watch your footing. About 15 minutes later, you'll hear, then see Twin Falls, then come upon Twin Falls Bridge.

You're now back in Lynn Canyon Park. And here you have two options. Either cross the bridge and make the final ascent to the parking lot on the west side of the creek. (And think about how before the bridge was built in 1930, the river had to be crossed on a large tree that had been felled across the falls.) Or you can take the steeper, slightly longer and more rewarding route along the east side of the canyon to the suspension bridge, and cross to where you started.

SEYMOUR RIVER & RICE LAKE LOOP

13

Distance: 7 km	Rating: Easy
Elevation gain: Minimal	Season: Year-round
High point: 350 metres	Topographical map:
Time needed: 2 hours	North Vancouver 92G/6
	Trail map: Page 75

Note: Dogs are not allowed in the Lower Seymour Conservation Reserve.

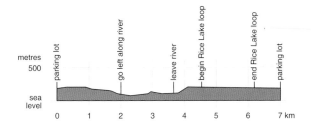

THOUGH NOT AS WELL KNOWN AS NEIGH-bouring Lynn Headwaters Regional and Lynn Canyon municipal parks, the Seymour Demonstration Forest is a great place to go when you're looking for a small hike with big variety.

Our route traverses second-growth forest to the banks of the Seymour River, where remnants of old homesteads and water pipes are visible, then up past towering old-growth trees and into the quiet tranquillity of the trails surrounding Rice Lake.

To get to the trailhead, take the Lillooet Road exit from the Upper Levels Highway. Follow Lillooet Road north, past Capilano College, past the cemetery and along the gravel road to the parking area.

Head to the northeast corner of the main parking area to find a gravel path that leads to a T-junction. Then go right to follow the Twin Bridges Trail to Seymour River.

On the way down this wide roadbed, where slopes have been laid bare by erosion, notice the different ways that sediment has been deposited—mostly it's flat layer on flat layer, but once in a while the strata are broken up by wild loops and whorls, likely created by eddies and currents flowing around a rock.

After 30 minutes or so, the trail arrives at the Twin Bridges—only one of which is still standing. Don't cross the bridge, but do pause for a view of Seymour River before heading north on

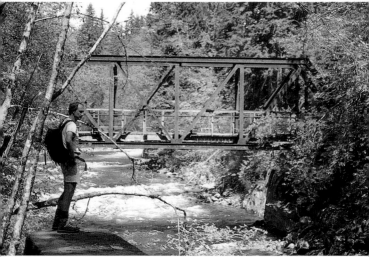

Seymour River and remaining Twin Bridge.

Fisherman's Trail flanking the river's west side. (Some fishing is allowed in the river. Consult regulations posted at the forest entrance before you cast a line.)

As the trail meanders along, keep a sharp eye off-trail for artifacts of the old water pipeline—cables, a rock-hewn tunnel and wooden support structures—and of the old homesteads that once stood along the river's edge. Old fence posts, gates, stone chimneys and foundations are still visible among the ferns, mosses and brush of the forest floor.

A leisurely 30 minutes of exploring brings you to a trail junction. Go left to follow the Homestead Trail. (The riverside trail does continue farther, but is often closed because of washouts and fallen trees.)

As the trail climbs upward, it passes several large Douglas firs—big and old, but still nowhere near the size and age of some of the real old-growth trees contained within the still-closed sections of the Seymour Watershed.

For years, the entire area was closed to the public, having been set aside for future water supply to the region. During World War II, mounted patrols guarded this area, to prevent acts of sabotage.

But in 1987, as demand for recreation space increased and with funding from the forest industry, the Greater Vancouver Regional District agreed to open a 5600-hectare area which is now called the Lower Seymour Conservation Reserve.

It is still considered future watershed and could be closed

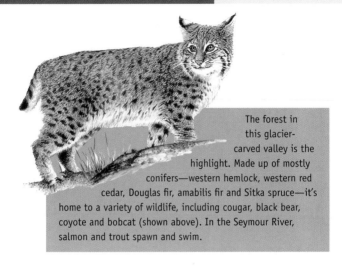

The forest in this glacier-carved valley is the highlight. Made up of mostly conifers—western hemlock, western red cedar, Douglas fir, amabilis fir and Sitka spruce—it's home to a variety of wildlife, including cougar, black bear, coyote and bobcat (shown above). In the Seymour River, salmon and trout spawn and swim.

to hikers if regional water consumption demands it. That's why this hidden treasure isn't a full-fledged park and why dogs aren't allowed. (Dogs can carry parasites that can affect the water supply.)

Twenty minutes of moderate huffing and puffing brings you back to the original trail junction. If you've had enough, simply retrace your steps to the parking lot. But, if you're up for 45 minutes or so of easy ambling, go right. A couple hundred metres farther, go left to take a trail that winds through a plantation of second-growth trees.

Cross over the roadway to the upper parking lot and follow the signs to Rice Lake. The lake wasn't always here, nor was it always surrounded by trees.

It is a manmade lake, created in the early 1900s by the Hastings Shingle Manufacturing Company, which operated a shingle bolt camp at the lakeside. Trees cut near Lynn Creek were transported by horse-wagon to a nearby mill, then by water flume to Rice Lake.

When the camp packed it in, the manmade lake became a reservoir to supply North Vancouver's drinking water. These days, it's a popular walking destination for locals and one of the few wheelchair-accessible hiking trails in the Lower Mainland. A small pier from which to catch some of the trout stocked in the lake is also wheelchair-accessible.

When you reach the start of the Rice Lake Loop Trail, go either right or left as the moment moves you. The loop itself takes only about 20 minutes to complete. By including

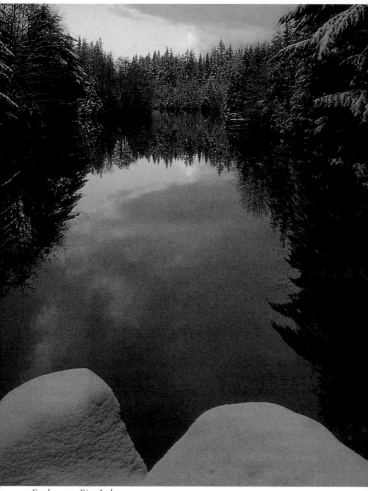

Fresh snow, Rice Lake.

the Forest Ecology Loop Trail, you can add another 10 to 15 minutes of exploration while finding out more about how forest managers manage forests.

Rice Lake is the perfect place to be on a rain-soaked day. While less-hardy folks hunker down indoors where it's warm, stuffy and dry, foul-weather walkers get to savour the lake and forest at its sweet-scented, tranquil best.

Then just follow the loop trail out, back to the parking lot.

MOUNT SEYMOUR

Distance: 8 km

Elevation gain: 450 m

High point: 1455 m

Time needed: 4–5 hours

Rating: Moderate

Season: July to October

Topographical map:
    North Vancouver 92G/6

Trail map: Page 75

Note: Dogs must be leashed.

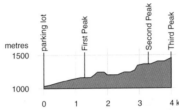

B IG MOUNTAIN VIEWS, SUBALPINE MEADOWS and easy access make Mount Seymour one of the most popular hiking destinations in the Lower Mainland. For that reason, expect lots of company on the trail.

Although there is a plethora of routes, ranging from a 15-minute jaunt to Dinkey Peak to a 13-hour overnight epic to Elsay Lake, the most trammelled trail is that to Mount Seymour itself, a three-peak experience.

We'll get to the trailhead in a moment, but first a word of caution. Although the access to Seymour's summits is relatively easy, the terrain can be extremely rugged—cliffs drop without warning and gullies can lead to precipitous dangerous drainages. The weather is also notoriously fickle on Seymour, changing from sunny and warm to cold, windy and cloud-socked in minutes.

Each year, hikers get lost on Seymour. The lucky ones get out cold and a bit worse for wear. But others have been seriously injured or died. Don't underestimate the mountain. Be prepared. (See page 14 for hiking essentials.)

To get to the trailhead, take the Mount Seymour exit off the Upper Levels Highway (the third exit on the North Vancouver side of the Second Narrows bridge) and bear right to turn onto the Mount Seymour Parkway. At Mount Seymour Road, turn left and follow it to the very top.

A BC Parks sign at the northwest corner of the parking lot is the starting point. Grab a Mount Seymour Provincial Park brochure/map and head north along the signposted trail. At the trail junction, go straight to take the narrowish trail that

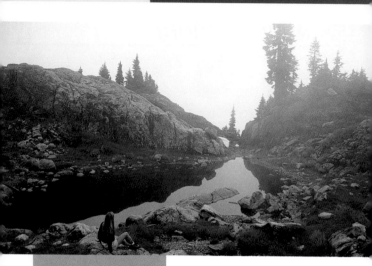

Even in less than perfect conditions, Mount Seymour has a unique beauty.

runs to the left of the chairlift. For about 40 minutes, the trail runs through subalpine meadows dotted with pondlets, alpine fir and wildflowers. Where the trail meets the Manning ski run, stay left and uphill along the rocky way for a couple of hundred metres, then follow the trail that leads down to the meadow and Sugar Bowl Pond on the left. From here, the trail clambers up a steepish section to reach the first real viewpoint of the hike at Brockton Point.

Although side-trails poke off to the right, the views from here on the main trail are just as grand. To the east are the greeny-blue waters of Indian Arm and the forested slopes of Eagle Ridge. To the north is the first peak of Mount Seymour. At times, rock climbers can be seen straddling its clefts and protrusions.

Early hikers used to start at sea level to climb Seymour. And although other North Shore mountains such as Grouse, Goat and Crown were climbed in the early 1890s, and logging roads have existed on Seymour's lower slopes since 1880, the first ascent of Seymour wasn't made until 1908 when members of the BC Mountaineering Club reached its 1455-metre summit.

In 1929, the Alpine Club of Canada made the first ski trip of the area and became involved in seeing Seymour preserved as parkland. The club leased 1000 acres from the provincial government, built trails and a cabin. Usage by both skiers and hikers increased as the years went by, but it wasn't until 1936 that Mount Seymour Provincial Park came into being.

From Brockton Point, there is a side-trail leading to the summit of First Peak, which is also known as Pump Peak. But we'll stay on the main trail and follow it down past a great view of Mount Baker and into more meadows. In summer, they're dotted with a variety of wildflowers and bugs. In autumn, the meadows are gloriously bug-free and filled with deep russets, glowing oranges and brilliant yellows of the fading fall foliage.

The trail crosses a couple of small creeks as it twists and turns. Numerous side-trails spill off; be sure to follow the bright orange diamonds to stay on track.

Soon, you'll come to a junction. Bear left to zig and zag up the east side of the First Peak, around tangled roots and past chunks of boulder. (Right goes on to Elsay Lake.) Eventually, the trail clambers into a rocky pass with views of First Peak dead ahead. Not much farther is the height of the ridge and, 10 to 15 minutes later, the First Peak.

A quick scramble to the top brings views all around, as well as gray jays looking for tidbits. For many people, this spot is the turnaround point, because of the weather or just because the day feels full enough.

If you want to continue to the third and final summit of Mount Seymour, the Second Peak is worth at least a water break. To continue, return to the main trail and drop steeply about 100 metres down into a notch between the two peaks.

The trail to the third summit drops steeply—about 100 metres down—into a notch. On reaching the bottom, you'll have to clamber back up to a rise, then up and down a minor hiccup of rock to reach a minor summit with the main peak in plain view. A bit more steep scrambling brings you to the true summit at 1455 metres. And in clear weather views of a virtual sea of mountains that stretch as far west as Sky Pilot, as far north as Mount Garibaldi, as far east as Golden Ears and as far south as Mounts Baker and Rainier.

Take a break, have some lunch and enjoy the scenery of Seymour. The mountain, by the way, as well as the river, an inlet, a lake arm and a city are all named after Frederick Seymour, who was the governor of BC from 1864 to 1869. His term of office came to an ignominious end when he died of acute alcoholism aboard *HMS Sparrowhawk*.

When you're ready to head back, retrace your steps carefully.

15 DOG MOUNTAIN

Distance: 6 km	Season: June to October
Elevation gain: Minimal	Topographical map:
High point: 1050 m	North Vancouver 92G/6
Time needed: 2 hours	Trail map: Page 75
Rating: Easy	Note: Dogs must be leashed.

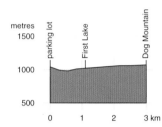

P OOR DOG MOUNTAIN. OVERWHELMED BY the three peaks of Mount Seymour and overlooked by many hikers as an unpedigreed perch not worthy of their attentions, it is in fact the perfect destination in a number of ways.

Because of its easy terrain, it's a great first hike for kids whose legs can't always manage high subalpine destinations. It's also good for adult neophyte hikers, for seasoned hikers who want a quick summer hike after work and for older folks. Heck, my 68-year-old mum accompanied me on one outing with no problems, except that I couldn't get her to tear herself away from the views, chipmunks and gray jays up top.

To get to the trailhead, take the Mount Seymour exit off the Upper Levels Highway and bear right to get onto the Mount Seymour Parkway. At Mount Seymour Road, turn left and follow it to the very top.

A BC Parks sign at the northwest corner of the parking lot is the starting point. From it, follow a wide gravel path north about 25 metres to a signpost with a map. Go left to follow the trail to First Lake and Dog Mountain.

Immediately, the trail enters the cool of the forest. Good-sized mountain hemlock and yellow cedar tower above the trail while at ground level are ferns, mosses and blueberry bushes. (In late summer and early autumn, when berries drip from their branches, be sure to make lots of anti-bear noise.)

The trail gently descends along a stretch that can include some rocky and root-tangled bits. It then undulates up and

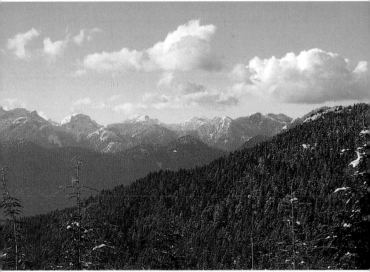

Dog Mountain (foreground), after snowfall.

down in a happy tail-wagging way for 15 to 20 minutes. Soon after, the trail levels into subalpine meadow and trickles down to first Lake.

In July, it's bug-o-rama here. But from August on, the cooler temperatures keep mosquitoes and no-see-ums under control. With luck, delicate sky-blue dragonflies will still be flitting along the shore. While it may look quite innocent, these are usually the male of the species cruising for a mate. Take a moment and you'll see them poke around lakeside vegetation, looking for females, which only visit water habitat to mate or lay eggs. Occasionally, a male dragonfly may stumble across another male and engage in a brief bout of wrestling. Then, they cruise on.

Dragonflies are such fascinating creatures that there are people who have made these insects and their behaviour a hobby. In BC, there are about 80 species of dragonfly and

Douglas squirrels chatter and scold from nearby tree branches, essentially trying to chase you from their territory. Watch for the azure flutter of a passing Steller's jay, the forest guardian who issues a throaty squawk to alert other animals to the presence of predators, such as owls, raccoons and people.

damselfly (a smaller, slimmer cousin). They are among the oldest known insects, dating as far back as 300 million years.

Unfortunately, the lifespan of a single dragonfly is at best 10 weeks. Enjoy them while you can. Continue along the trail into the forest. Fifteen minutes further are more small pondlets on either side of the trail. Then it's back to the world of the forest.

Because it's a short amble, you can take time to enjoy the minutiae that are often overlooked on more strenuous outings. Check out some of the weird saprophytic plants that flourish in the dank humus of the forest floor. These plants are conspicuous by their lack of green. That's because they don't contain chlorophyll, the substance that allows most plants to convert sunlight and waterbound nutrients to food through photosynthesis.

Saprophytes make their meals from dead and decaying vegetation—the stuff of which most forest floors are made. Here, you'll likely see the reddish-brown lances of pinedrops, which can grow thigh-high. (The Okanagan people called them 'coyote's arrow.') Look also for the nodding pinky-yellow pinesap, which can grow shin-high.

As you near your destination, the forest thins and the trail passes over a couple of exposed rocky outcrops, including one that you may want to slide down, seated. At a handpainted sign noting the way back to the parking lot, stay left to emerge onto the prominent bluffs of Dog Mountain. (Okay, it's not really a mountain, but 'Dog Bluffs' probably just didn't excite its namers.)

To the northwest are great mountain views. Lynn Peak is the undulating bump in the foreground; Coliseum Mountain is the grand, rippled peak farther north. The outlines of Crown and Camel mountains can be made out in the distance. Directly below is the Seymour River, slithering towards Burrard Inlet.

At the south end of the bluffs are remnants of two old cabins. Rotting timbers and rusted metal bits are all that remain of the former Greater Vancouver Water District lookouts. Views to the south are the vast sprawl of Greater Vancouver and, on clear days, some of the Gulf and San Juan islands.

Take a break to enjoy the views, a snack or lunch—which the resident gray jays and northwestern chipmunks will undoubtedly want to share—then retrace your steps to the parking lot.

BADEN-POWELL TRAIL

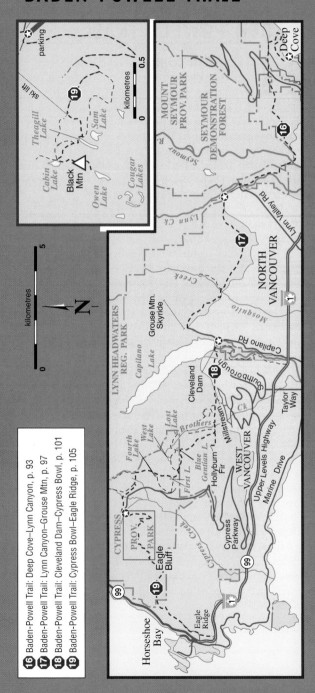

16 Baden-Powell Trail: Deep Cove–Lynn Canyon, p. 93
17 Baden-Powell Trail: Lynn Canyon–Grouse Mtn., p. 97
18 Baden-Powell Trail: Cleveland Dam–Cypress Bowl, p. 101
19 Baden-Powell Trail: Cypress Bowl–Eagle Ridge, p. 105

BADEN-POWELL TRAIL

HIGH IN THE NORTH SHORE MOUNTAINS, rambling through groves of old-growth cedar, meandering around mountain lakes and traversing steep slopes is a trail that's a well-kept secret.

People may have read or heard of it. They may have seen roadside signs marking its access points. They may even have walked a section. But not many non-hikers realize that the Baden-Powell Trail is, in fact, a magnificent 48-kilometre route stretching from Deep Cove in North Vancouver to just shy of Horseshoe Bay in West Vancouver.

Thanks for the Baden-Powell Trail go to the 1000 Boy Scouts and Girl Guides who hacked and cleared brush, built bridges and steps, burned slash and hammered markers in 1971. The trail—named after Boy Scout founder Robert Stephenson Smyth, Lord Baden-Powell—was a project to mark BC's 100th birthday. The idea was to provide hikers with the wilderness experience, right in their backyards.

These days, parts of the trail are quite literally in our backyards; housing subdivisions have encroached farther into the forested slopes. In other parts, the trail is a paved road, hardly what its builders had in mind.

Although it is possible to cover the entire distance in about 20 hours, not many folks will opt for such a power-hike. Fortunately, the Baden-Powell Trail has many access points, many connecting with secondary trails at Seymour, Grouse and Hollyburn, that allow you to complete a circuit of your own design.

I've broken the trail into four sections, each 10 to 15 kilometres long. Section one covers Deep Cove to Lynn Canyon, section two covers Lynn Canyon to Grouse Mountain (see page 97), section three covers Cleveland Dam to Cypress Bowl (see page 101), and section four covers Cypress Bowl to Eagle Ridge (see page 105).

Transportation should be arranged for both ends of the hike. Bicycles can be dropped off at the trail-ends beforehand. Some trail-ends and trailheads are served by public transit. Have a friend pick you up, or arrange to leave a second vehicle at the trail's end.

DEEP COVE TO LYNN CANYON 16

Distance: 12 km

Elevation gain: 405 m

High point: 425 m

Time needed: 5 hours

Rating: Easy

Season: Year-round

Topographical map:
   North Vancouver 92G/6
   & Port Coquitlam 92G/7

Trail map: Page 91

Note: Arrange for transportation at both ends. A 210 bus or 229 bus from Peters Road near Lynn Canyon will take you to the Phibbs Exchange. From there, catch the 212 Deep Cove bus back. For more information, call Translink at (604) 953-3333 or www.translink.bc.ca

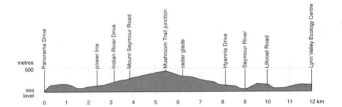

THE FIRST SECTION OF THE BADEN-POWELL Trail is neither the wildest nor the most urban of the bunch. On the plus side are beautiful forest groves and scenic river canyons; on the minus side are the occasional subdivision and paved road.

To get to the trailhead, mosey out to Deep Cove, driving either over the Second Narrows bridge and along the Dollarton Highway, or down the Mount Seymour Parkway if you're already on the North Shore. Just as downtown Deep Cove begins, you'll see Panorama Drive. Turn left and park in the public lots on your right.

The trail gets off to an unpromising start at its eastern end—the trailhead being literally squished between two houses on Panorama Drive. You'll feel as though you're wandering into someone's backyard as you head up the driveway just past 2501 Panorama, but not to worry, you're on the right trail.

Make note of the orange squares nailed to the trees at regular intervals: they are the trail markers you'll be following. (There are also white maps posted at crucial intersections along the trail to keep you on track.)

About 30 to 40 minutes into your hike, just before a bridge—built by Capilano College volunteers in 1981—is a

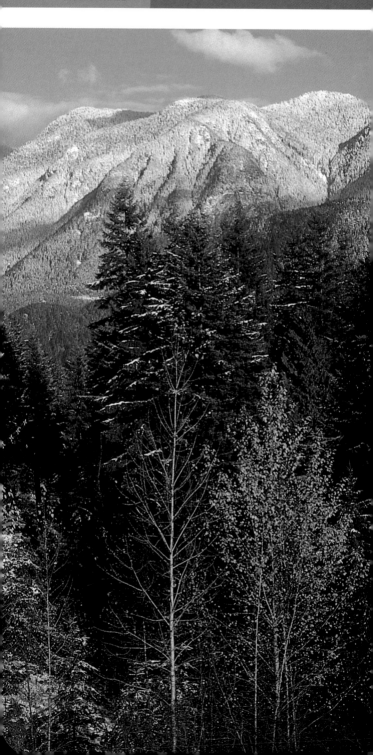

great big Douglas fir. How big? About 3.5 metres in diameter, big enough that it would take two 1.8-metre-tall people to wrap their arms around.

> The forest quickly takes over as soon as you hit the trail. Western hemlock and western red cedar replace houses and backyards and *voilà*, you're suddenly away from it all.

When you come to a clearing with a view of the power line, bear right into the forest again and arrive at a rocky bluff with views of Deep Cove, Belcarra and Burnaby Mountain. Farther along, just under a power pylon, is another grey granite massif with sightlines to Buntzen and Eagle ridges.

After soaking up the views, head eastward away from the water, then left about 10 metres from the power line on the continuing trail into the forest. The path will bring you a few minutes later to a dirt road, which you'll cross, bearing left for a few metres to pick up the trail again.

Eventually, you'll come to the pavement of Indian River Drive. When the trail was constructed, this road was dirt; now it's a concrete intrusion into the hiking psyche. Maybe it will be rerouted in the future; for the present, you will simply have to pound pavement westward for about 500 metres.

At the big water tank on the north side of the road, it's time to cross and pick up the forested trail again. Another 20 or 30 minutes of walking will bring you to the Mount Seymour Road—more pavement—which you'll cross carefully to pick up the trail on the other side.

Ambling along, you'll come to an intersection with the Old Buck Trail, named after the man who operated Buck's Logging in the early 1900s and who built this old logging route from Mount Seymour to Deep Cove Road. (A skid road continued to the waterline, where logs were then towed to nearby booming grounds.) Twenty years later, a forest fire raced up the flanks of Mount Seymour, and Buck's was out of business.

A bit farther is the Mushroom Trail. Here, take the left fork, which drops into a glade of big cedars and big cedar stumps. Continue to the intersection with the Good Samaritan Trail.

Now, the trail loses elevation as it descends toward the Seymour River. Although the going is easy, you'll need to pay close attention at the next trail intersection—about 30 minutes away. Here the only signs around both have horses on them. To the left is a brown sign with a horse. To the right is a

Fall foliage and snow on the Baden-Powell Trail.

silver-coloured horse marker. Follow the silver pony to avoid the subdivisions.

About 100 metres farther, where a hunk of rock protrudes, the trail splits again. Go right and prepare for another close encounter with civilization—Hyannis Drive. Cross the road and follow the trail down through a section that will once again make you feel as if you're wandering through backyards.

Soon, the trail joins with the path that runs along the east side of the Seymour River. Go left. A few minutes farther and—urban sprawl again. Do not cross the wooden bridge. Instead, take the trail heading down to the river and a metal bridge.

Under this span, the Seymour River thunders through a narrow gorge. From its headwaters at Loch Lomond, the Seymour River trickles about 11 kilometres southeast, picking up speed and volume as it is joined by hundreds of feeder creeks. The Seymour Dam has flooded about 7 kilometres of the old river valley, turning it into Seymour Lake, one of the reservoirs on which the Greater Vancouver area depends for drinking water.

With that in mind, look, smell and listen to the river. Then take a deep breath for a short steep grunt up stairs and trail. About the same time as the sounds of the Seymour River recede, the path levels into quiet forest, then crosses a concrete pipeline and emerges under a power line. (Those snow-capped peaks in the distance are Mount Seymour.)

At the next intersection, continue straight. A few minutes of easy walking brings you to the gravel of Lillooet Road. Cross it, then bear left for about 50 metres to pick up the continuation of the Baden-Powell Trail.

The sounds of Lynn Creek trickle through the trees as you head into the forest. At the next signpost with a map, follow the trail that leads directly downhill.

Go down, down, down to the boardwalk, over the marshy ground and to the water's edge. The trail meanders alongside the mist-draped creek through some muddy, wet and slippery sections, so watch your footing. About 15 minutes later, you'll hear, then see Twin Falls, then come upon Twin Falls Bridge.

You are now in Lynn Canyon Park. From here there's a final ascent to the parking lot along the canyon's east side and over the suspension bridge, where your parting views are of rapids rushing through the narrow gorge and a veil of waterfall tumbling down the canyon's west wall.

LYNN CANYON TO GROUSE MOUNTAIN

17

Distance: 10 km	Rating: Moderate
Elevation gain: 200 m	Season: Year-round
High point: 500 m	Topographical map:
Time needed: 4–5 hours	North Vancouver 92G/6
	Trail map: Page 91

Note: Arrange transportation for both ends. Bus 228 Lynn Valley or 229 Westlynn will take you to the starting point; bus 236 Lonsdale Quay or 232 Phibbs Exchange will bring you down from Grouse. For more information, call Translink at (604) 953-3333 or www.translink.bc.ca

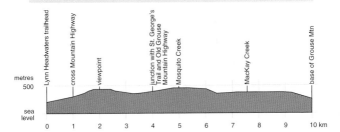

THE SECOND SECTION OF THE BADEN-Powell Trail features lovely forest groves and sparkling creeks, but also some inevitable backyard hiking thanks to urban sprawl.

We last left the Baden-Powell just as we crossed over the Lynn Canyon suspension bridge. If someone is driving you to the second trailhead, take the Upper Levels Highway to the Lynn Valley Road exit and head north. Follow the signs to Lynn Headwaters Regional (not Lynn Canyon) Park and park in the overflow lot closest to the park entrance.

Just across the road is the start of the trail proper (as opposed to the roadway portion of the BP Trail here). Where the signs and orange markers note the Baden-Powell Trail, head into the forest for a short steep scramble up a set of wooden stairs.

At the top, catch your breath and go left along an old skid road. Then, just 100 metres later—before the fence and houses—bear right and up again.

The trail winds away from urban encroachment and enters a glade of second-growth forest with such a magical feel that I half-expected to see Bambi romping among the trees.

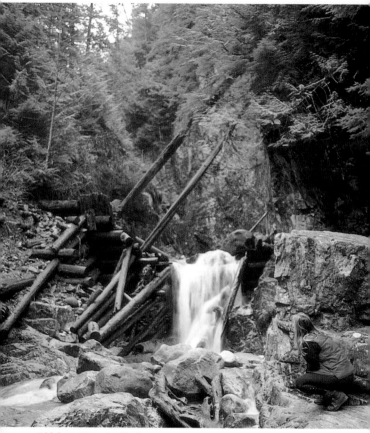

Old dam, Mosquito Creek.

In 15 to 20 minutes, the trail arrives at the small debris-choked Thames Creek and, a bit farther, some blowdown. One triumvirate of hemlocks has fallen directly over the trail. Another cluster of six leans over, awaiting their final rest from the next windstorm.

In another 10 to 15 minutes, the trail meets Mountain Highway. Cross for a short steep uphill grunt over trail that needs some restoration work. Some mountain bikers—not all, just some—have ignored the ethics of trail riding while hammering downward and have cut switchbacks, smashed steps and gouged ruts in the trail, causing erosion and sometimes precarious footing.

With not too much slipping and sliding, though, you'll come to the top, where the trail flattens out and winds through evidence of an old forest fire. Huge, blackened trunks and stumps crouch within a forest of big red alder trees.

Just 15 to 20 minutes later is the first viewpoint, with Burrard Inlet in the foreground, and the cities of Vancouver, Richmond and Delta sprawling southward.

Then it's back among the trees and into what I dubbed 'The Spirit Forest.' Here, numerous cedar snags stand like silent sentinels, phantoms

Two old cedar snags stand nearby, limbless and wizened. The size of the trunks—almost 2 metres in diameter—hint at their earlier majesty when they would have stood up to 40 metres tall, covered in thick red bark, draped with fragrant green boughs.

of the old-growth forest that once lived here. They're crooked and decrepit, but still lingering, poignant reminders of what once was.

From here the trail drops to Kilmer Creek, which you'll cross into a sun-dappled forest. Twenty minutes later is a major trail intersection: downhill leads to St. Georges, uphill to Mount Fromme, and straight ahead to the Baden-Powell Trail. Nearby is a bench on which to sit and ponder, perhaps munch a trailside snack and take in the views of Stanley Park, Point Grey and the ocean beyond.

Back on the trail again, cross a small nameless creek and, a few minutes later, listen for the rushing and rumblings of a larger waterway—Mosquito Creek. Where the trail forks, stay right, towards the two green water tanks. Pass them, following the signs to the creek. Cross the creek by stepping stones.

Civilization now intrudes for about 20 minutes of walking. When you see the house with the orange metal roof, head uphill (following the orange arrow). At the top of a short grunt is another view of the city. Go right and uphill—naturally—and, at the next intersection, right again. The road first swings back then continues uphill, traversing a rakishly sloping hillside.

The long, slow grind will feel worth it, though, when you come to MacKay Creek, with its beautifully steep drainage, its waters plummeting into a narrow ravine. A plank bridge used to cross MacKay, but during the fall of 1995, record rainfall turned the creek into a torrent of water. The bridge was washed away, houses downslope were flooded and the creekbed was scoured down to bedrock. Downed trees still litter the waterway.

So, until repair work is done both by Mother Nature and volunteer trailbuilders, take care when scrambling down and up the steepish sides to cross the creek. (Don't do it at all if the water is running high.)

After crossing another tributary of MacKay, the trail

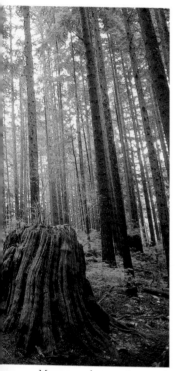

Moss-covered stump in second-growth forest.

meets with the first of two trails heading upslope to the old BC Mountaineering Club cabin, used as a base for climbing and hunting trips to Dome, Dam and Crown mountains. In an article called 'Cabins, Camps and Climbs: 1907 to 1911,' club member Frank Smith recalls some of the tribulations faced by early women hikers and climbers: Forced by the laws of polite society to wear a skirt reaching to her heels and clothed above in some form of blouse with long sleeves and high neck, the picture was completed by a pair of heavy nailed boots peeping from below the skirt…. Of course, the skirt had to be discarded at the first opportunity, bringing into view a pair of bloomers which ballooned out from the waist and draped over the knees. A more unsuit-able garment for the local bush could hardly be conceived. It simply invited every snag to grab it, with disastrous results.

As well, the ferry company that conveyed passengers from Vancouver to the North Shore had a strict rule forbidding any women passengers to board while attired in bloomers. On one occasion, notes Smith, 'an unfortunate bloomer girl had to send word across and have some relative come over with a skirt to enable her to get home.'

Amble merrily and skirtlessly along for another 20 minutes, past more monster snags and give thanks that change is eternal. Before you know it, you'll be at the parking lot at the base of Grouse Mountain.

CLEVELAND DAM
TO CYPRESS BOWL

18

Distance: 12 km	Rating: Moderate
Elevation gain: 565 m	Season: June to October
High point: 1065 m	Topographical map:
Time needed: 5 hours	North Vancouver 92G/6
	Trail map: Page 91

Note: Arrange transportation at both ends. Buses 232 and 236 Grouse Mountain will take you to the starting point, but there is no bus service from Cypress Bowl. For more information, call Translink at (604) 953-3333 or www.translink.bc.ca

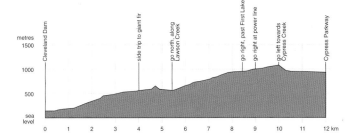

THE THIRD SECTION OF THE BADEN-Powell Trail may begin with urban sprawl, but it quickly ascends into the beautiful forest-cloaked slopes of Hollyburn Mountain and expansive views.

We last left the Baden-Powell at the Grouse Mountain Skyride. And so, technically, that's where we should pick it up. But, because the next 2 kilometres of 'trail' is actually the pavement of Nancy Greene Way, make the starting point Cleveland Dam.

To get to the trailhead, head for Capilano Road just east of the dividing line between West Vancouver and North Vancouver. Follow Capilano Road north and look for the green and yellow GVRD Parks signs noting the entrance to the Cleveland Dam parking area.

From the top of the dam are northward views of The Lions and of Capilano Lake, which supplies water to the Greater Vancouver area. Once through the dam, the lake waters plunge 90 metres to the Capilano River below. Having taken in the power of the nature, walk west across the dam and look for the Baden-Powell's entrance into the forest—a trail that heads up and to the right.

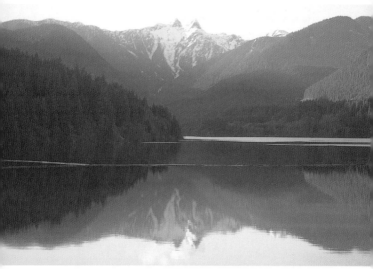

The Lions and Capilano Lake, seen from Cleveland Dam.

A few minutes later, just before a chainlink fence, turn left into the trees. And about 100 metres later, where the trail forks, go left and up again.

During the next 30 to 45 minutes you must literally hike through backyards where the only views are of swingsets, barbecues and sundecks. The only old-growth you're likely to see is the moss on the power poles; the only wildlife a noisy sheltie just before you hit St. Giles Road.

Finally, the path comes to a power substation where Millstream and Craigmohr roads intersect. Cross the road and head into the trees. About 10 minutes in, the trail splits; left goes to Millstream and more suburbia, right trundles under the power line along the Baden-Powell Trail.

A bit farther is another junction. Go left. In 20 to 30 minutes the trail meets with the Forestry Heritage Walk with its markers. Stick with the familiar orange squares. The trail dips into the canyon of Brothers Creek, a trough carved out of the bedrock by ancient glaciers. The west canyon wall is granite, which pushed to the surface about 100 million years ago; the east wall is basalt or lava, which crystallized about 32 million years ago.

Stop on the bridge to ponder the geological history of the area and savour the view of the creek's lovely waterfall. Notice also the big Douglas fir, amabilis fir, Pacific yew and western hemlock that stand here. In the 1920s, loggers took only the more valuable western red cedar to make into shakes and shingles.

A short slog up the opposite canyon wall brings you to a T-junction. The right fork goes to Lost Lake. We, however, will take the left fork, which, in a few minutes, meets the intersection with the Skyline Trail.

> The Hollyburn fir has the greatest recorded circumference of any Douglas fir still standing. It is estimated to be about 1100 years old. In girth, it measures about 10 metres—big enough that it would take more than five 1.8-metre-tall tree-huggers to hug it.

The Baden-Powell Trail actually continues to the right, along Lawson Creek. But we're going left for a 45-minute side-trip for a visit with one of the biggest trees in Canada—the Hollyburn fir.

Follow the Skyline Trail under the power lines. At the bridge that crosses Lawson Creek is a stately western red cedar—the first hint of bigger, older trees yet to come.

Once out of the ravine, the trail passes through a sanctuary of huge old snags and remnant stumps, some as big as 6 metres in girth. Rufous-sided towhees, woodpeckers and ravens—the Hollyburn Symphony Orchestra, as I like to think of them—warble, rattle and caw a requiem to the former forest giants.

After a bit of hiking reverie, the trail joins the power line again. Pass a small creek and watch the power poles on the left for the one with a silver-coloured '6' on it. Just opposite, a trail cuts right and into the forest. Follow the orange markers for about 20 to 30 minutes and you'll arrive at the Hollyburn fir, all 43.7 skyward metres of it.

As you look up to where the branches disappear into the mist, imagine walking in an entire forest of these giants, instead of the stumps and smaller second-growth now here. With that thought in mind, head back to Skyline Trail, turning left to retrace your steps back to the connection with the Baden-Powell Trail.

From here the Baden-Powell heads uphill, but it's not that steep an angle. Not that you'd notice: you'll be too busy taking in the sights of cedar boughs weighed down by new growth, of tiny mosses, mushrooms or wildflowers and the occasional glimpse of Lawson Creek.

About 45 minutes along, the trail passes the intersection with a trail to Blue Gentian Lake, and, a few minutes farther, a major intersection with multiple trails.

In May and June, snow may still linger here. But it's usually hard-packed enough to walk on without significant difficulty. With the cross-country ski operations shut down from May to

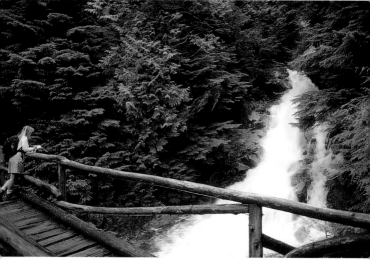

Lawson Creek, Baden-Powell Trail.

October, you can continue on the Baden-Powell as it heads up along the old ski hill to join with the Grand National ski trail.

If a substantial amount of snow still lingers, you'll have to cut your hike short and bear left for Hollyburn Lodge and beyond to the parking lot. But, if the snowpack has dwindled enough to allow safe crossing of two tributaries of Cypress Creek, continue uphill on the Baden-Powell as if toward Hollyburn Peak.

The trail looks down on First Lake and Hollyburn Lodge, passes the warming hut and Fourth Lake and comes to a crucial intersection. Go left here to continue on the Baden-Powell to Cypress Bowl (right goes to the peak).

Soon comes the first creek over which you'll cross via a beautiful wooden bridge that master trailbuilder Halvor Lunden built—with the help of fellow hikers and BC Parks.

Between here and the Cypress Bowl parking lot, the trail winds through groves of old-growth trees.

CYPRESS BOWL TO EAGLE RIDGE

Distance: 12 km	Rating: Moderate
Elevation gain: 340 m	Season: July to October
High point: 1215 m	Topographical map:
Time needed: 6 hours	North Vancouver 92G/6
	Trail map: Page 91

Note: Arrange transportation at both ends. Buses serve neither the Cypress Bowl nor the Eagleridge interchange.

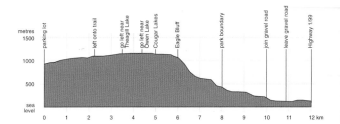

W E LAST LEFT THE BADEN-POWELL TRAIL at the Cypress downhill ski area parking lot, and that's where we'll pick it up. From the Upper Levels Highway, take the Cypress Provincial Park turnoff. To get to the trailhead, drive up the Cypress Parkway to the downhill ski area. Park in either lot and head for the trail signs near the ski area buildings. Because of development in the ski area, changes are coming for this chunk of the Baden-Powell trail. At present, you can still start at the northwest corner of the parking lot and wind your way up the switchbacks to the top of the Black Chair. But the plan is to start rerouting the trail in 2004 or 2005. The new trail is slated to start from the little wooden bridge on the Yew Lake Loop Trail, then climb through the forest to the Fork ski run and, finally, join an old "shortcut trail" to Cabin Lake.

From here you can see evidence of the logging that has taken place in the park, and imagine the controversy it caused. In the late 1930s, much of the Cypress Valley was slated for logging by the Heaps Timber Company of Los Angeles, California. Local residents were not happy, nor were skiers who'd built facilities and lodges on Hollyburn in the 1920s. Political pressure eventually forced the provincial government to exchange timber leases on Vancouver Island and, in 1944,

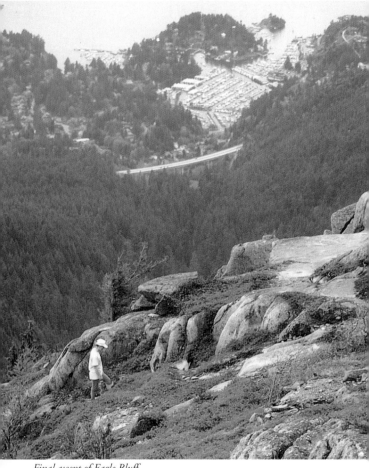

Final ascent of Eagle Bluff.

to set aside Cypress Bowl as a park reserve—but not before 40 hectares had already been logged.

Thirty years later, controversy reared its head again when Alpine Outdoor Recreation Resources won a bid to develop a ski resort that included a 7000-house subdivision, parking space for 5000 cars and an artificial lake. In less than two years, the company logged more than 10 million board feet of timber. After public outcry, logging was halted and an interim plan was drawn up. But controversy erupted again when more than 120 hectares of municipal timber was cut and sold.

Strangely enough, there is a new controversy over the cutting of trees in Cypress. A private company, which operates the downhill and cross-country facilities, wants to expand its operations. Under the company's proposed plan, more than 43 hectares of old-growth trees could be cut.

It's something to ponder as you head for the trees directly behind the chairlift's huge concrete counterweight and look for the orange squares that indicate the way down. A few minutes later is a trail junction. Straight ahead is part of the Black Mountain Loop Trail, but we'll go right around the northern end of Theagill Lake.

About 15 minutes of walking brings you to Cabin Lake, where you can brave the chilly waters for a swim if you're so inclined. From here, the trail heads up and south for another 10 minutes or so. And then you'll find yourself—at 1217 metres—on the lower of Black Mountain's two summits. (The north summit is a mere 7 metres higher.)

Once you've soaked up the 360° views, follow the markers down to Owen Lake and, a bit farther, Cougar Lakes. Then it's on to Eagle Bluff. The trail heads back into the forest again and gradually down.

Follow the orange squares and aluminum plates, which lead to Eagle Bluff for 30 to 40 minutes. At the junction with the Do-Nut Rock trail, bear left until you reach the rocky bluff.

You'll know when you've arrived. The views seem somehow even more stunning than those you've seen higher up. Maybe it's the steepness of the bluff; maybe it's Eagle and Whyte lakes shimmering below; maybe it's the antics of the little forest robber barons, otherwise known as gray jays or whiskeyjacks. In any case, this spot is the perfect place to sit, contemplate and eat lunch.

When you're ready to continue, head down the lower reaches of the bluff, following the orange arrows painted on the rock. This part of the trail is **very** steep, so you may feel happier descending on your bum at times. I say: if it feels good, do it.

Twenty to 30 minutes of knee-knackering descent brings you to a big rock slide. Pick your way down and across, following the orange markings and orange flags through the talus. Watch your footing—many an ankle has been twisted here and there are still another couple of hours to the trail's end.

With the rock slide behind, the trail hits dirt again. The path meanders along a kinder, gentler slope through Douglas fir and western hemlock, past titanic granite boulders, back and forth across Whyte Creek, eventually meeting with a trail intersection. Stay left, towards the Upper Levels Highway, just as the sign says.

Another 30 to 40 minutes of walking along a wide access road through mixed deciduous and coniferous forest brings you

Summit views, mountain lakes and pockets of old-growth forest make the fourth section of the Baden-Powell Trail both the most unique and the most spectacular of all.

to a view point—and, glory hallelujah—a rough-hewn bench. Take a few minutes to rest your tired feet and watch sailboats and powerboats zip across the channel between West Vancouver and Bowen Island. The long, rude *blaaaat* of a ferry departing Horseshoe Bay tells you you're almost at the trail's end.

Twenty minutes later is a small pond and a funky trail sign. Continue straight through for one final uphill grunt. Once at the top, it's only a few minutes to the Eagleridge parking lot.

Note: The future of this last section of the Baden-Powell Trail is in flux because of improvements to be made to the Sea to Sky Highway. If the provincial government decides to build a four-lane highway here, the trail will have to be rerouted. If a tunnel is built, the trail is not likely to be affected.

WEST VANCOUVER

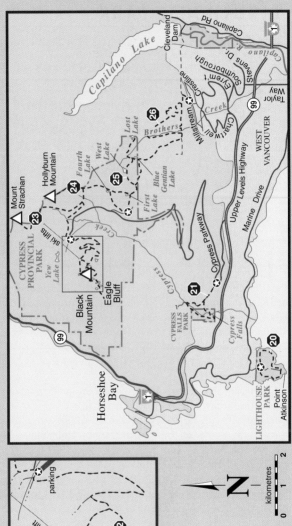

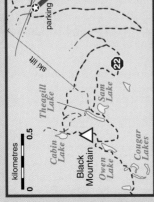

20 Lighthouse Park, p. 110
21 Cypress Falls, p. 114
22 Black Mountain, p. 118
23 Mount Strachan, p. 122
24 Hollyburn Peak, p. 126
25 Hollyburn Ridge, p. 130
26 Brothers Creek Loop, p. 135

20 LIGHTHOUSE PARK

Distance: 6 km

Elevation gain: Minimal

High point: 115 m

Time needed: 2 hours

Rating: Easy

Season: Year-round

Topographical map:
    North Vancouver 92G/6

Trail map: Page 109

Note: Dogs must be leashed.

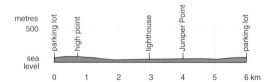

T HANKS FOR THIS TREASURE IS SELF-
evident in its name: Lighthouse Park. The first light
house—a picturesque little wooden structure, as it was
then described in a local newspaper, was built on Point Atkinson
in 1874. Not long after, 75 hectares of land surrounding the
beacon were set aside as a reserve by the federal government. In
1910, the land was leased first to North Vancouver and then,
in 1912, to West Vancouver when it became a full-fledged city.
The land is still owned by the federal government, but is leased
to West Van for $1 a year.

There are many trails to traipse in the park. You can
head straight down the main road to the lighthouse. Or you
can head off with map in hand and see things most folks
miss—things such as some of the largest Douglas firs in
Greater Vancouver.

To get to the trailhead, follow Marine Drive in West
Vancouver for almost 10 kilometres, past Caulfeild Cove.
Watch on the left for the Lighthouse Park sign, and turn left
on Beacon Lane. Follow the road to the right, and park in
the lot.

The starting point for our roughly circular route lies at the
top of the parking lot. Stop for a look at the information board,
then scoot past the yellow gate and look on the left for a small
post with a white #1 painted on top. Go left.

Follow the trail up to a red and white fire hydrant. Now,
go right. About 50 metres farther is a side-trail that will take
you to the park's summit at 115 metres. If you happened to
be looking towards English Bay in say, 1792, you might have
spotted Captain George Vancouver, the man who gave this

Lighthouse Park.

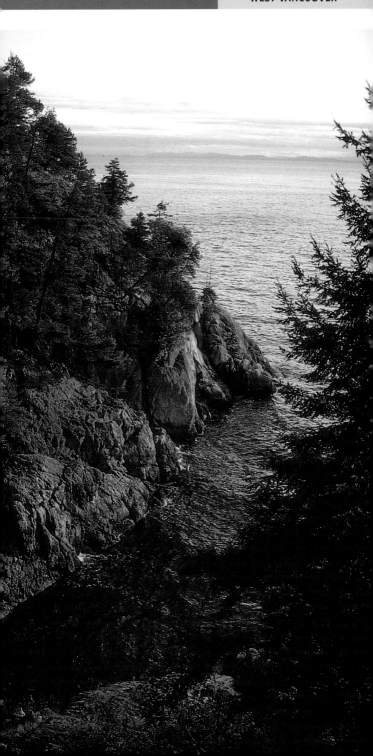

piece of land its geographical name, and wrote the following in his journal:

> On the northern side the rugged snowy barrier, whose base we had now nearly approached, rose very abruptly and was only protected from the wash of the sea by a very narrow border of low land. By seven o'clock we had reached the NW point of the channel...this I called Point Atkinson.

After the summit, retrace your steps to the main trail and continue east, watching for a trail on the right, just next to a fallen moss-covered log. (If you come to a rocky outcrop on the left, you've gone too far.)

Follow the trail down to a junction. Then go right, following the white arrow-shaped markers. As the trail descends through a grove of western red cedar and Douglas fir, your jaw may also drop in awe.

Some of the bigger firs are 67 metres tall and 6 metres around. In human terms, that's more than 37 1.8-metre-tall men standing on one another's heads. (With another four similarly tall folks at the base, touching outstretched fingertip-to-fingertip in a circle.)

Burn scars on some trees attest to the wildfires that have swept through the forest in the past. Still, many of the Douglas firs in the park are between 400 and 550 years of age. When these trees were seedlings, Christopher Columbus was just a baby himself.

Eventually, the trail reaches a junction. Go left for the moment and take any one of the many side-trails that lead to viewpoints at the water's edge. This area is also one of the best in the Lower Mainland to see the granodiorite of the Coast Mountain Plutonic Complex—or, in non-geological terms, the granite that forms much of the rugged mountain scenery in southwestern BC. About 100 million years ago, molten granitic rock, formed deep within the Earth's crust, rose slowly then solidified. Then, during the last 40 million years, overlying rock was eroded to reveal the great smooth tongues of granite.

These wave-washed outcrops are a great place to break for lunch, and for contemplation.

Retrace your steps to the junction from where you came and head west. A switchbacky section brings you to another beautiful grove of big trees and a junction. Bear left and follow the trail to a collection of cabins and the lighthouse.

These days, the lighthouse is automated, but it wasn't always. Lighthouse keepers and their families once lived here, and what a remote and isolated spot it was.

On one stormy night in 1883, word reached the settlement of Moodyville (later to become North Vancouver)

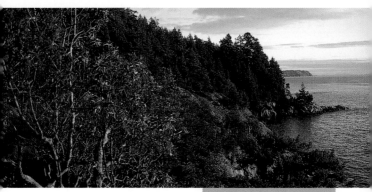

that the wife of lighthouse keeper Walter Erwin had become seriously ill. Despite the hazards involved in such a storm-wreaked journey, Emily Susan Branscombe, or as she is referred to in an archival account, 'Mrs. John Peabody Patterson, a beloved and practical woman,' volunteered to go to the lighthouse and care for the ailing woman (whose first name has been lost to history).

The shores of West Vancouver hide a tiny peninsular pocket of wilderness. The western hemlocks, western red cedars and Douglas firs here have never been logged. And, in one of the highest-priced real-estate markets in the country, the land has never been developed or subdivided.

In 1883, the north shore of Burrard Inlet was a rocky terrain of trail-less forest, an impenetrable tangle of undergrowth, impassable swamp, and unfordable stream; access to the lighthouse was by water only. A gale was raging in English Bay; the masters of the paddlewheel tugboats counselled delay, the risk was great and dusk was falling. The Squamish Indian Chinalset offered his dugout canoe and together they paddled into the black of the storm and night, reaching the lighthouse as dawn broke.

After a nod of recognition for the heroic, or should we say heroinic, feat, continue west towards Jackpine Point with its views of Bowen Island. Side-trails spill off the main trail as it makes its way back to the parking lot. Each has its own merits. Which paths you follow and which you leave for another outing are up to you. At some point, include a wander to Juniper Point, where rock-climbers hone their skills and where bald eagles nest.

Then just follow the signs east to the main parking lot where you began.

21 CYPRESS FALLS

Distance: 6 km

Elevation gain: 130 m

High point: 300 m

Time needed: 2 hours

Rating: Easy

Season: Year-round

Topographical map:
North Vancouver 92G/6

Trail map: Page 109

Note: Dogs must be leashed.

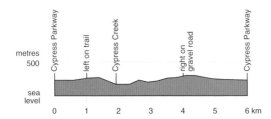

EVEN ON THE NORTH SHORE, THERE IS NO season in which you must hang up your beloved hiking boots. Winter is the perfect time to explore all the shorter, lower-level hikes that seem suited to the shorter, cooler, wetter and often windier days. Just shrug off the unwelcoming elements, invest in some good raingear and head for the treasures to be discovered on a winter's trail.

Cypress Falls Park is such a gem. This area is not the Cypress Provincial Park familiar to most folks, although it is close by. Cypress Falls Park is a small West Vancouver municipal park filled with waterfalls, old-growth trees and sylvan sensibilities.

Although trails are accessible from three different locations, allowing you to spend as little as 30 minutes or as long as two hours poking around, our jaunt begins just off Woodgreen Place.

Follow the Upper Levels Highway to the exit for Caulfeild and Woodgreen Drive. Go right on Woodgreen Drive past Woodcrest Road. Then turn right on Woodgreen Place. There are two parking areas—the first few spots are near the tennis courts, but there's an old gravel pit just a few metres farther with more parking.

From the parking area, head toward the trees to find the main trail. Go left and follow the trail as it climbs slowly upward. At a fork, stay straight ahead.

Soon the trail will bring you to a rustic wood bridge, Cypress Creek and the Lower Falls.

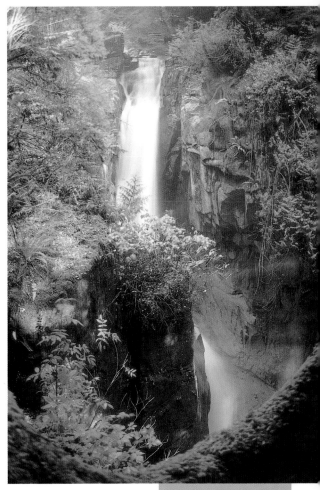

For a different view of the falls, head back up the trail just to the top of the rise and follow a side-trail that scoots to the left and down. From here, you see the falls from the falling-end as the water tumbles into a chasm of granite ledges decorated with mist-happy ferns.

The water squeezes through a narrow rock chute to ricochet off a rock ledge in a crescendo of white spray, while slow-moving plumes of mist rise from below.

Continue along the trail as it shadows the creek until it meets with the main trail. Turn right and, a couple of hundred metres later, follow the path as it juts to the left. After a few minutes, the trail splits into a three-pronged fork. The left turn leads to a clearing; the right back to the lower falls. We'll go straight.

Almost immediately the trail passes through a small grove of big trees. These Douglas firs, estimated to be about 400 years old, survived logging earlier in the century, and still bear the bark-blackened scars of a forest fire long ago. The tallest of these Douglas firs reaches about 60 metres, about the same height as the Sun Tower, a Vancouver heritage building on Beatty Street.

With such surrounding loveliness, it's hard to imagine that only 60-some years ago, the area suffered from the effects of 'indiscriminate logging practices.' John Davidson, BC's first provincial botanist and then president of the Vancouver Natural History Society, delivered a scathing rebuke of local forest companies in a 1924 address to the society:

> A few years ago, a company started a mill on Hollyburn Ridge, part of which drains into Cypress Creek.... The Spring freshets turned the otherwise beautiful creek into a roaring, rushing, turbulent torrent, breaking its banks, washing out roads and paths and depositing a deep layer of sand and gravel over the lawns and gardens of residents.

> ...We cannot overestimate the value of a reliable source of cold, fresh water, furnished by slowly melting snows, percolating through the sand, gravelly soil and cool shady forests to the water intakes; Vancouver is in an enviable position in this respect. When the citizens of Vancouver realize the necessity of the trees on the mountain slopes for the maintenance of this supply, they will not tolerate any interference with the timber or any part of the watershed.

Unfortunately, Davidson was proved wrong. Logging was allowed in the 1930s in the Cypress Bowl area; its scars are still easily visible. And proposals are once again being made by the private company that operates the downhill and cross-country ski areas, to cut more trees (some old-growth) for more ski runs and facilities.

It's something to consider as you continue along the trail for another few minutes to the next fork. Go right, towards the creek and cross a small wooden bridge over a feeder stream. (You should still be on the west side of the main creek.)

Just on the other side of the bridge is a prominence that affords a lovely view of Cypress Creek as it tumbles through a moss- and fern-covered gorge, past a couple of slowly decomposing wood leviathans that slid downslope long ago.

As the trail continues through the forest, the sound of upper

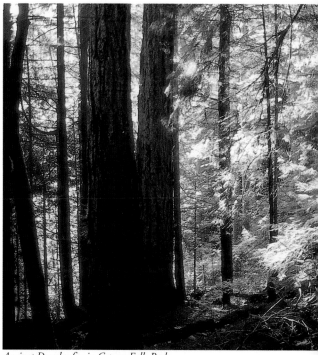

Ancient Douglas firs in Cypress Falls Park.

falls becomes audible. Soon, a graceful cascade of white water appears, plummeting 10 metres into one pool, sweeping over rock and into another pool, then trundling on as a creek once more. The lushness of the surrounding moss, ferns and under-storey gives the upper falls an almost tropical look. You half expect to see some scantily clad Polynesian maiden treading water in the lagoon-like pools below (though in this case, she'd be voted 'swimmer most likely to develop hypothermia').

Once you've soaked up the reverie, retrace your steps to the Lower Falls, and then to the parking area.

22 BLACK MOUNTAIN

Distance: 11 km	Rating: Moderate
Elevation gain: 300 m	Season: June to October
High point: 1215 m	Topographical map:
Time needed: 5 hours	North Vancouver 92G/6
	Trail map: Page 109

Note: Dogs must be leashed.

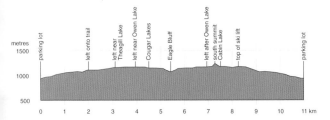

SPARKLING SUBALPINE LAKES, WINDING forest footpaths and some of the most magnificent views ever seen from the North Shore are the rewards for a hike that demands only modest efforts.

From the Upper Levels Highway, take the Cypress Provincial Park turnoff. Drive up the Cypress Parkway to the downhill ski area, park your car and head for the trail signs near the ski area buildings.

Because of development in the ski area, changes are coming for the first part of your hike. At present, you can still start at the northwest corner of the parking lot and wind your way up the old logging road to one hairpin bend, continue to the next junction, go left to continue to a second hairpin bend.

Follow the faded orange ribbons to a narrow path through the forest, quiet and fragrant with the scent of fallen evergreen needles. The trail passes some small brackish ponds and, later, a big boulder rockfall. Here, the trail can seem vague, but it does head uphill. Just look for the neon orange square in the near distance.

After about 30 minutes, the shimmer of a lake peeks through the trees on the left. Not much farther, the trail intersects with the Black Mountain Loop Trail.

However, if you happen to hit this trail after the changes, you'll need to take a different start. The new route is slated to start from the little wooden bridge on the Yew Lake Loop Trail, then climb through the forest to the Fork ski run and, finally,

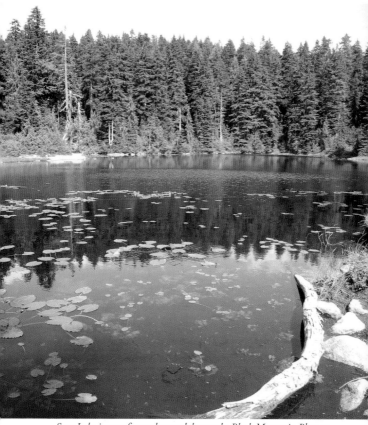

Sam Lake is one of several pretty lakes on the Black Mountain Plateau.

join an old "shortcut trail," which will bring you to a junction at a section of boardwalk. Go left to follow the trail down to Theagill Lake and Sam Lake, the first two of the many tarns of Black Mountain plateau.

Others follow. Owen Lakes and Cougar Lakes; each will call out, tempting you to stop. Go ahead. Just keep track of time and remember you've got another three hours or so to go.

Continue to Eagle Bluff, following the trail back into the forest as it occasionally dips down. Follow the orange squares and metal plates for about 30 to 40 minutes, staying left at the junction with the Do-Nut Rock trail.

When you finally arrive at the bluff, you'll know it. Even though the sights south are mostly urban and suburban sprawl, the view is indescribably vast and thus remarkable. As well, you can see across to the peaks of the Sunshine Coast and far out to the San Juan and Gulf islands.

The Black Mountain Plateau is the perfect outdoor classroom to learn a bit more about the concepts of biogeoclimatic zones, site associations and other vegetation-related stuff that scientists use to classify a particular place. Although all the terminology can seem daunting, think of it as a long, detailed address, like John Doe's suite, The Cypress Building, Westmount Neighbourhood, West Vancouver, BC, Canada, North America.

In the case of this address, though, we'll work backwards from ecosection to vegetation site associations. Of the 72 ecosections in BC, the Black Mountain Plateau lies within the Southern Pacific Ranges Ecosection, a vast, rugged area of more than 1 million hectares that stretches from the North Shore farther north to past Powell Lake.

Because the type of vegetation within an ecosection varies according to elevation and climate, the next part of the address is a biogeoclimatic zone. Of the 14 such zones in BC, Black Mountain Plateau lies within one called the Mountain Hemlock, where the most common trees are yellow cedar, amabilis fir and, of course, mountain hemlock.

Things get more specific when we move to site associations. The Black Mountain Plateau is home to the HmBa-Mountain Heather site association, because of the predominance of mountain hemlock, amabilis fir (also known as balsam fir, thus the 'Ba' of the 'HmBa' name) and mountain heather.

It's important to remember that describing a place in such terms is not merely a pedantic scientific exercise. The descriptions also play a pivotal role in determining which areas will be designated as parks. Under the Protected Areas Strategy, the province has promised to protect 12 percent of the land base from development. Although it would be easier to designate hectares of rock and ice, the 12 percent must also include undisturbed areas such as low-elevation old-growth forests, which are rare in some parts of the province.

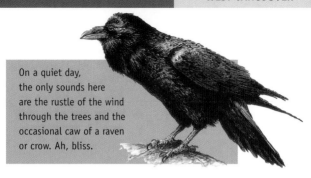

On a quiet day, the only sounds here are the rustle of the wind through the trees and the occasional caw of a raven or crow. Ah, bliss.

The wide-open tumble of rock is the perfect place to stop for lunch. Savour the views while you eat your sandwich. And watch hard-core hikers come up the trail from Horseshoe Bay—a steep seven-hour trek.

After lunch, return along the trail you came in on. But at Owen Lake take the left leg of the Black Mountain Loop Trail up to the south summit for northward views of The Lions and the Tantalus Range. Maybe stop for a moment of reflection on the origin of the mountain's name—after a forest fire more than 100 years ago that left tree-covered slopes little more than standing charcoal. You may also decide to hike a few minutes more to Cabin Lake—a great spot for swimming when it's warm. (Note: Cabin Lake was once named Paradise Lake. Apparently all the names at Cypress were changed in the 1970s by BC Parks, for some unknown reason. If you know, send me a note.)

Then it's on to whichever trail you came up on—the ski runs and logging road before changes, or the new route after changes. Either way, it's about 25 minutes down to the parking lot at Cypress Bowl.

23 MOUNT STRACHAN

Distance: 10 km

Elevation gain: 528 m

High point: 1445 m

Time needed: 6 hours

Rating: Moderate

Season: July to October

Topographical maps:
  North Vancouver 92G/6

Trail map: Page 109

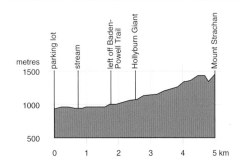

MOST FOLKS WHO HIT THE HEIGHTS OF Mount Strachan in Cypress Provincial Park do the summer ski-run slog and trudge up a barren rocky road to the south summit.

But there's a much more enjoyable way to the top, through old-growth forest, subalpine meadows and along a trail used in the late 1890s and early 1900s by hikers and mountaineers. This is Strachan by way of the western slopes of Hollyburn Mountain, a pretty alternative. (The Old Strachan Trail fell into disuse after other routes were created, and was only recently rediscovered.)

From the Upper Levels Highway, take the Cypress Provincial Park turnoff. To get to the trailhead, drive up the Cypress Parkway to the downhill ski area. Park in either lot, then head for the BC Parks map and information signboard. From here, head right, towards the trees to the Baden-Powell Trail sign and follow it east.

Immediately, you're in a forest grove. About 15 minutes later is a makeshift crossing over a small creek. You'll want to start checking out the trees. Only a few minutes past the creek, immediately following a marshy bit of trail, is part of the Road Stand: five significant yellow cedars ranging in age from 270 to 1075 years. (Two of the trees stand almost directly opposite one another on the trail; the others are farther downslope.)

Another 10 minutes brings another creek to cross. Master trailbuilder Halvor Lunden and the Hollyburn Trekkers who've

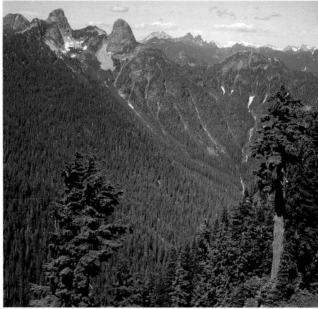

Views from the summit of Mount Strachan include The Lions.

adopted this part of the Baden-Powell want to build a bridge here. But because of the controversy involving expansion of the downhill ski area, the bridge has been put on hold.

After gaining a bit of elevation, the trail comes to an earlier bridge that Halvor built—well, actually, designed, built and installed with the help of fellow hikers and BC Parks. If you were to cross Halvor's bridge, you'd connect with the trail to Hollyburn Peak. We, however, will go left, onto the Old Strachan Trail.

Halvor rediscovered the trail a few years back and set about clearing and marking it, along with members of the BC Mountaineering Club. The trail, he says, was commonly used as long as 100 years ago, when hikers and mountaineers followed this route to The Lions and other peaks on the far western Howe Sound Crest. Traverse in their footsteps, essentially retracing the lower trail but at a higher elevation. Relax, this is the scenic route where you get to revel in the coolness provided by the old forest.

After about 30 minutes, right where a big rock sits in the middle of the trail, look left of the trail for two strips of orange tape, tied about 5 metres apart. There, you'll see the ancient yellow cedar known as the Hollyburn Giant. Although its top was broken off long ago, it still stands impressive at more

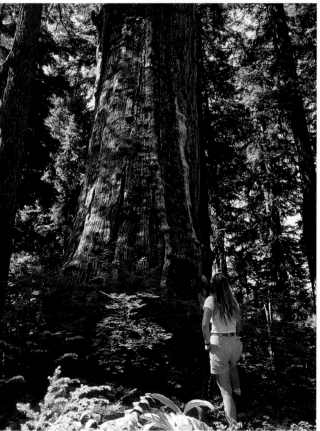

The awesome Hollyburn Giant is worth a closer look.

than 20 metres in height and 10 metres in girth. The tree is estimated to be more than 1000 years old, which means that when it was a seedling, the Vikings were raiding Britain, France, Spain and other parts of Europe and Leif the 'Lucky' Ericsson first stumbled across North America on the shores of Newfoundland.

Although the Hollyburn Giant's future was once in question because of a proposed expansion plan by the private company that operates the downhill ski facilities, the latest plans would not remove the tree nor any of the other old growth in this area.

And now, back to the trail. Continue along the path as it leads from forest to subalpine meadow, which in summer can be a veritable bug-o-rama—mosquitoes, blackflies, no-see-ums.

Unpleasant, yes, but it gives you incentive to keep moving.

You may also encounter a bit of blowdown and leftover snowdrifts on the way up. Just plod on to a point where the trail forks, then follow the tine

> In early summer, the trail is lined with the white blooms of queen's cup and delicate sprays of foamflower.

that goes up and left, past the 'Danger: Ski Area Boundary' sign. The forest trail shadows the ski run and is much cooler and more scenic.

Fifteen to 20 minutes of wandering through pink and white mountain heathers brings you to a big rock into open meadow. Scramble down, then follow an old trail as it rambles through meadow, then steeply up to the summit of Strachan. If you're comfortable with a rough ascent, continue on. Otherwise, head left onto the ski run and follow the markers on a more gradual rise to the top.

The steeper route passes the site of a plane crash. A metal plaque attached to a tree tells the whole story: 'These are the remains of a Canadian Air Forces T-33 trainer which crashed on 23 November 1963, killing two. Do not take anything.'

If you've wandered over to look at the debris of this tragedy, retrace your steps to an orange marker pointing the way to the top. For at least 30 minutes the trail slogs through muck, roots and bugs. Once you hit the open rocky bluffs, it's not much farther to the top.

The 360° views from the south summit make it all worthwhile. To the west is Howe Sound and the Sechelt Peninsula, to the northeast are mountains as far as the eye can see, including Grouse, Seymour and Coliseum, and to the north is a spectacular view of The Lions.

Before the arrival of non-Natives, these twin spires were known to the Coast Salish people as Checheyohee, The Two Sisters. (For the legend of The Two Sisters, see page 159.) Pauline Johnson's book *Legends of Vancouver* tells us how Chief Joe Capilano spoke of the Sisters in 1911:

> On the mountain crest the Chief's daughters can be seen wrapped in the suns, the snows, the stars of all seasons, for they have stood in this high place for thousands of years, and will stand for thousands of years to come, guarding the peace of the Pacific Coast and the quiet of Capilano Canyon.

After some quiet contemplation on the summit, simply retrace your steps back down. Or opt for a faster retreat along the ski runs by staying right of the storage shed on top and following the green tapes down through blueberry bush.

24 HOLLYBURN PEAK

Distance: 8 km

Elevation gain: 440 m

High point: 1325 m

Time needed: 4 hours

Rating: Moderate

Season: July to October

Topographical map:
 North Vancouver 92G/6

Trail map: Page 109

Note: Dogs must be leashed.

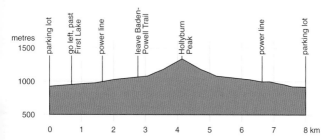

S OMETIMES, YOU WAIT UNTIL THE LAST minute before deciding to go on a hike. Sometimes, it's because the weather starts off ugly then gets better. Sometimes, you just can't drag yourself out of bed in time for an early morning start.

But at some point you decide you just have to get out and up in the mountains, even if there's only a few hours of daylight left. And that's the perfect time to do this hike to the top of Hollyburn Mountain.

Our route starts at the Hollyburn Ridge cross-country ski area. To get there, take the Cypress Provincial Park turnoff from the Upper Levels Highway, and head up Cypress Parkway. Near the top, watch for the turnoff to the cross-country area and follow it right. Then park.

In autumn, it can be rather cool up top, even on the sunniest of days. Be sure to include a wool sweater or fleece jacket and long pants—and raingear—in your daypack. You may end up not using them, but if the weather changes suddenly, you'll be happy you packed a couple of extra kilos.

From the lot, head up the wide path alongside the forest to the power line. After 10 to 15 minutes, the trail level reaches the height of the saddle. Stop to catch your breath, have a sip of water and soak up the views of the Gulf of Georgia, the Gulf Islands and Vancouver Island.

Then continue east under the power line, passing Fourth Lake on your left. Typical subalpine meadows provide a

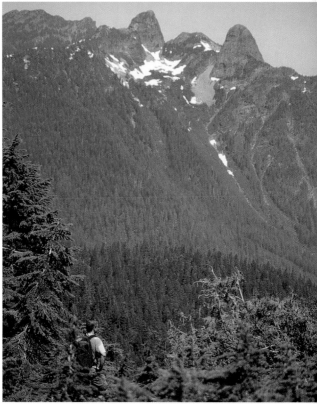

View of The Lions from Hollyburn Peak.

variety of sights and smells in the wildflowers, shrubs and stunted trees. In September and October, the place is resplendent in the warm shades of autumn.

The south-facing slope of Hollyburn Mountain differs significantly from the steep exposed rock of the north face. The reason? Glaciers. Between 15,000 and 25,000 years ago, vast sheets of ice moved south through the Coast Range, undercutting high points and fracturing rock where the ice made

One word of warning about all this lush vegetation: in autumn, when succulent blueberries abound, so do black bears. Keep an alert eye out; bears can become oblivious to just about everything when hoovering berries. And make noise on the trail—talk, sing, whistle—to let bears know where you are, so they can scoot in the other direction. (For more bear sense, see page 21.)

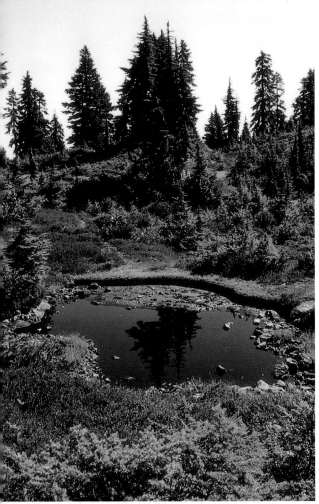

Heather Lakes area, below Hollyburn Peak.

contact with the mountain. On the south slopes, though, glaciers deposited 'till'—the silt, sand, gravel and boulders picked up and ground by the advancing ice sheet.

Where the trail meets the warming hut, turn left and follow the trail uphill through the forest and meadow. From time to time, other trails cross and spill off from the main path, but just continue on and up. Another 45 minutes or so will bring you to the perfect spot for a rest stop. A few metres off the main trail, to the right, is a bench with views of Grouse, Dam, Goat and

Crown mountains just across the Capilano Valley.

After a break, continue your upward journey. Fifteen to 20 minutes of steady hiking brings you out of the trees and into a open, rocky area dotted with small ponds. (In summer, they're essentially mosquito-breeding pits. Bring bug spray.)

Continue north to a steepish scramble up a rocky prominence. Here, you might consider how the 1930 party who made the first ascent by 'saddle pony' may have covered that bit of ground. Then continue on—there's still a few more vertical metres to cover.

After a few minutes more of zigzagging, the trail reaches the 1325-metre top: Hollyburn Peak with its panoramic view. Directly north is Mount Strachan, and farther beyond, the twin spires of The Lions. In the near east are Grouse, Goat and Crown mountains, and a bit farther distant, the aptly named Cathedral Mountain.

Thousands, perhaps millions, of hikers have enjoyed their lunches on this peak since early in the century when Hollyburn was a favourite destination of such groups as the BC Mountaineering Club and the Varsity Outdoor Club. As you munch away amid a sea of peaks and valleys, you'll likely be approached by descendants of the northwestern chipmunks and gray jays who insisted on sharing your predecessors' food. Whether it's genetics or practice, be warned: some of these little alpine robber barons are exceedingly bold and may try to carry off an entire sandwich, not just a proffered crumb.

The polished rock on which you're sitting is different from the rock at the parking lot level. There, it's hornblende granodiorite—some of the North Shore mountains' oldest rock. But the peak of Hollyburn is a pendant of banded amphibolite and metasedimentary rocks belonging to the Bowen Island Group. Or, in non-technical terms, it is a remnant of younger rock material either spewed from a nearby volcano or deposited by river or ocean as sediments, then squeezed by pressure and temperature into metamorphic rock. A similar 'pendant' exists in Mount Gardner on Bowen Island (see page 143).

On your return from Hollyburn Peak, you can head back down the same route, or, from the warming hut, continue south towards Hollyburn Lodge and First Lake for a look at a bit of human history before heading west once again to the parking lot.

25 HOLLYBURN RIDGE

Distance: Up to 10 km

Elevation gain: 250 m

High point: 1000 m

Time needed: Up to 3 hours

Rating: Easy

Season: June to October

Topographical map:
        North Vancouver 92G/6

Trail map: Page 109

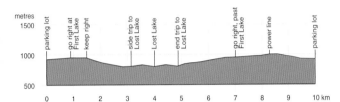

HIGH ON HOLLYBURN RIDGE IS AN elaborate system of trails used since the 1920s and '30s by folks of all kinds. Hikers leave few historical traces, but a wealth of cultural legacies have been left behind by generations of cross-country and downhill skiers. Although some people might find the remnants of human activity disturbing in such a mountainside setting, age has given the relics an air of quaintness.

To get to the trailhead, follow the Upper Levels Highway to West Vancouver and take exit #8 to Cypress Provincial Park. Follow the Cypress Parkway up and take the turnoff east to the cross-country ski area parking lot.

From the trailhead sign, follow a wide path heading toward the forest, under the power lines. On a clear day, there are views of the city, the ocean and distant Gulf and San Juan islands. Follow the path straight ahead where a cross-country ski sign notes the direction to Hollyburn Lodge.

Most of the wildflowers growing along the wide-open road have faded by the end of summer, but in autumn a few remnant lupines, fireweed and valerian remain, lending small swatches of colour to the forest of green. Succulent blueberries dangle from bushes everywhere. Have a few—just to taste—but leave the rest for the birds, bears and other animals that depend on them for sustenance.

Within 10 minutes, the trail passes alongside a moose-rack adorned cabin, the first of a handful of old cabins in the park. During the 1920s, '30s and '40s, ferries used to transport hikers

Dawn Hanna, Blue Gentian Lake.

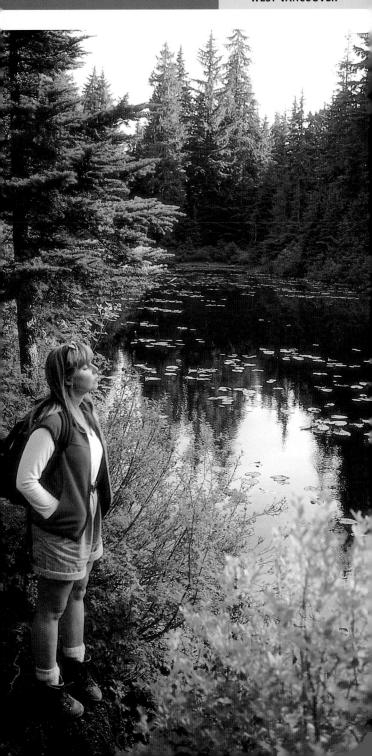

This hike takes in reminders of pioneer ski days as well as ancient landscapes. From the sadly dilapidated Hollyburn Lodge to huge old-growth trees, an early fall hike on Hollyburn Ridge is the perfect way to bid summer adieu.

and skiers from Vancouver to the shores of West Vancouver. After slogging all the way uphill, they stayed at the cabins for what was then a wilderness weekend.

Continue past other cabins towards the red building just ahead—Hollyburn Lodge. Built in 1926 from lumber salvaged from an old mill, the lodge has hosted many an event over the years. Unfortunately, the lodge and some of the cabins may not stand much longer. According to a 1995 report, the building had been allowed to fall into such disrepair by the private company that used to operate the downhill and cross-country facilities, that it may be 'too far gone for effective renovation.' While some people consider the lodge a heritage building and want to see it preserved, the commission recommended that the company be allowed to tear down the lodge and construct a reproduction.

The front of the lodge looks out onto First Lake, a small subalpine tarn. There, a signpost shows your location. Continue along the shore past the Ranger Station and the municipal cabin area and across the bridge/dam.

A few metres farther is a four-way junction with a signpost and map. Go right to follow part of the Baden-Powell Trail or, as it's known in winter, the Grand National ski trail. Heading downhill, the trail passes another couple of cabins—the memorable Doghouse among them. Just beyond the second cabin, on the right side of the trail, is a big old western hemlock measuring about 5 metres in circumference. Although much of the lower ridge was logged early this century, some old trees—and occasional groves of first-growth—escaped the axe and saw.

At the next junction, bear right to continue down the Baden-Powell/Grand National, following the sign that points the way to the old West Lake Lodge. Although this is usually a wide road, by summer's end only a narrow trail exists among all the ferns, berry bushes and other mountain shrubbery. Stay on the trail as it descends, curves, then heads briefly uphill before emerging to a clearing.

Rusting bits of an old ski lift constructed of wood, old car wheels and axles still remain. There are also good southeasterly views of North Vancouver, Burnaby and other parts of the

Lower Mainland. Descend carefully on the loose rock of the trail to a lower bluff with good views east of Goat and Crown mountains and the Camel tucked behind Grouse.

Just below this clearing stood the old West Lake Lodge. It was built in 1933 on the shores of West Lake, but when the lake was designated as a watershed for West Vancouver a few years later, the lodge and surrounding cabins were dismantled and, piece by piece, moved here. A later lodge was built in 1948, but in 1986, it burned to the ground.

From the bluff, go left and downhill, keeping left again at the next junction. Watch carefully for the trail breaking off to the left. (A sign points to Blue Gentian Lake, but it's hidden among the foliage and is not easily visible when coming from the north.)

Follow the boardwalk east past another old ski hill remnant to the next junction about five minutes distant. Here, go left and follow the trail into the forest. Five minutes farther, the trail forks. Go left again, following the sign that points the way to Blue Gentian Lake. Stoney Creek trickles through the canyon on the left as the trail descends through rooty, rough terrain.

About 10 minutes later, as you near a trail junction, come the first views of the tiny subalpine lake. In summer and sometimes early fall, the shores are carpeted with the lake's namesake—a lovely violet-blue flower known as the king gentian. It's believed to be the richest population in the Lower Mainland of this relatively uncommon bloom.

While you take a break here, consider your next steps. It's possible to meander farther east, crossing Stoney and Brothers creeks and descending through some beautiful old-growth groves to Lost Lake. The mountains there have a silent, wild, ancient feel to them. It's no surprise that this area of the park is where northern spotted owls have been sighted. The owls, an endangered species, need 800 to 1000 hectares of old-growth forest in which to live.

But the route to Lost Lake is recommended only for experienced hikers because of the poor condition of the trail and the potential for getting, well, lost. If your hiking experience is minimal or the weather threatening, return instead to the trail junction and head north, following the sign that points to West Lake.

After five to 10 minutes is a T-junction. Go right to West Lake. (Left retraces your steps back to the old ski run.) The trail continues along the creek on level ground, then up a root-tangled section before emerging to West Lake.

It's possible to follow a trail around part of the lake, but eventually you'll want to go left from the dam and follow the way to Hollyburn Lodge, which is pointed out by an old wooden sign way up a tree. Another 10 to 15 minutes brings you to another trail junction. In winter, you can ski or snowshoe through towering yellow cedars up Mobraaten Trail, but in summer and fall the route is choked with bushes. Go straight, taking the right fork of the Jack Pratt Trail and at the top of the steep rise you'll find yourself in familiar terrain where Jack Pratt joins the Baden-Powell/Grand National. Regain the four-way junction higher up.

If you're still up for more scenic strolling, continue straight ahead to a viewpoint overlooking First Lake and Hollyburn Lodge. Trundle downhill to where the trail intersects with the Sitzmark Trail and continue straight ahead, following the signs pointing to the 'Warming Hut.'

A short stiff uphill grunt leads to the hut, used to warm cross-country skiers in winter. From under the power line are views east to Grouse, Seymour and peaks beyond. Directly behind the hut is a quartet of little lakes and the path to Hollyburn Peak. But when you've soaked in the views and are ready to head home, simply head west and follow the wide path under the power line down to the parking lot. Splendid views of Point Grey, Georgia Strait and distant islands bid you goodbye.

BROTHERS CREEK LOOP

26

Distance: 7 km

Elevation gain: 350 m

High point: 700 m

Time needed: 4 hours

Rating: Moderate

Season: March to November

Topographical map:
    North Vancouver 92G/6

Trail map: Page 109

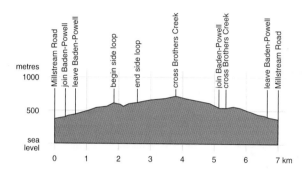

T UCKED HIGH ON THE SLOPES OF WEST
        Vancouver is a remnant grove of big western red cedars
        that must have a guardian angel. Having escaped
the axes and saws of early loggers, they stand tall and stately,
despite the lack of formal protection. (The giants stand on
West Vancouver municipal land. It has yet to be designated
as parkland.)

The toughest part of the hike may be finding the way to the
trailhead through the maze of streets in the British Properties.
Follow Taylor Way north under the Upper Levels Highway,
then bear left on Southborough Drive. At Highland Drive, bear
left again and follow the road as it snakes uphill to Eyremont
Drive, where you'll turn left. At Crestline, go right, then shortly
after at Henlow, go left. This brings you to Millstream Road.
Turn right and a couple of hundred metres farther is the yellow
gate that marks the start of the trail.

Don't park in front of the gate. And use common sense about
parking on the roadside. Remember, this is a neighbourhood,
not a parking lot.

Trundle past the gate along a wide path. The parallel logs
underfoot betray the path's origins as the support for a unique
locomotive known as a Walking Dudley, used here between
1908 and 1913. Now, the way also serves as a fire access road.
After 10 minutes of walking, the Baden-Powell Trail intersects.
Go left.

A few hundred metres farther, the trail forks again.

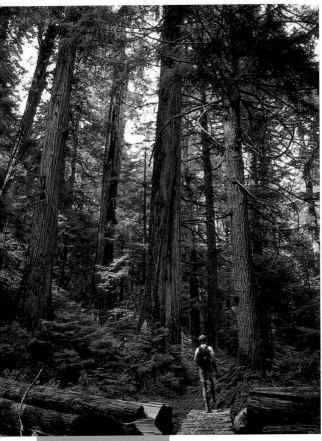

On the hike up Brothers Creek, you'll see big trees—from snags to living giants, Douglas fir and western red cedar—as well as waterfalls and remnants of early logging.

Go right. Soon, you'll see the stone foundation and other remnants of the boilerhouse of a steam sawmill built in 1912 and abandoned in 1913.

Continue upward and onward for 20 minutes to the intersection with the Crossover Trail. For a shorter, two-hour winter trip, the turnaround point is here. (Just bear left through second-growth forest, cross the bridge at Brothers Creek, follow the trail down to the Baden-Powell, head east to the wide road and back to the gate.)

For the full four-hour tour, continue along the old skid road as it zigzags through the trees, passing through a part of the forest once logged of its cedars to make shingles. Seventy years ago, an old incline cable railway ran where you now walk. After 15 minutes of hiking, the trail takes a sharp hairpin turn. Don't follow it yet, but go straight, then right to take a worthwhile side-trip to see the Candelabra fir.

Follow the bright yellow markers downslope for about 10 minutes, past massive stumps and some blowdown, and suddenly, the giant tree is suddenly before you—more than 9 metres around, more than 60 metres tall, despite the elegantly broken tops that give it its name. (The tree is about the same height as the old Sun Tower building on Beatty Street in downtown Vancouver.)

Although this Douglas fir is now one of many sizable dead snags in the area, a living giant still stands just a few minutes farther downhill. This tree, also a Douglas fir, measures 43 metres in height, about the same as a 10-storey building, and 8.5 metres in girth.

After taking it all in, return to the main trail and follow it uphill as it winds its way through old-growth western hemlock, amabilis fir and, soon after, a beautiful grove of western red cedars—some almost 8 metres around.

Some of the taller trees poking bare-limbed above the understorey appear to be dead snags, but telltale branchlets of green foliage attest to their living state. For 20 wonderful minutes, the grove continues until you hear the rushing waters of Brothers Creek.

History records that this stream was once called Sisters Creek, and was believed—mistakenly—to have its headwaters at the base of The Sisters peaks, now called The Lions. No note has been made as to why the sex change took place.

Unless some trail maintenance has been done, you may have to wriggle under or walk around a big hunk of blowdown to come to a clearing. On a tree above is a weatherworn sign pointing the way to Lost Lake, but it's a hike best saved for another day. Instead, stop for lunch, a snack and a rest before crossing the creek and returning downhill.

A wooden bridge once spanned the creek; now, however, you'll have to cross gingerly on stones. (Take special care during the high waters of spring.) Once on the other side, bear left at the stump. (Right goes to Blue Gentian Lake, another hike best saved for another day. See page 130.)

As the trail heads down, occasional glimpses can be had of two small waterfalls. Don't venture too near the cliffs—it's all too easy to slip and tumble a long, cold way down. Not much farther down the trail is another beautiful grove of cedars. Here, where the trail is steepish, and the rough-hewn

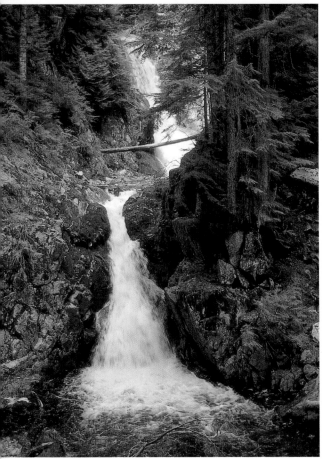

Upper Falls, Brothers Creek.

'stairs' are slippery, it's best to stop for a good long look at the surrounding marvels.

About 40 minutes downcreek is the intersection with the Crossover Trail. Take a peek at the bridge and the view, then continue straight for another 15 minutes or so until the trail intersects with the Baden-Powell. Go left and follow the path out of the forest, under the power line and down to a scenic bridge crossing Brothers Creek.

After a short steep section climbing out of the ravine, the trail meanders through second-growth forest punctuated with spiralling snags and slowly decaying stumps until it meets with the old skid road. From here, it's a short 10-minute amble to the yellow gate that marks the end of the road.

BOWEN & GAMBIER ISLANDS

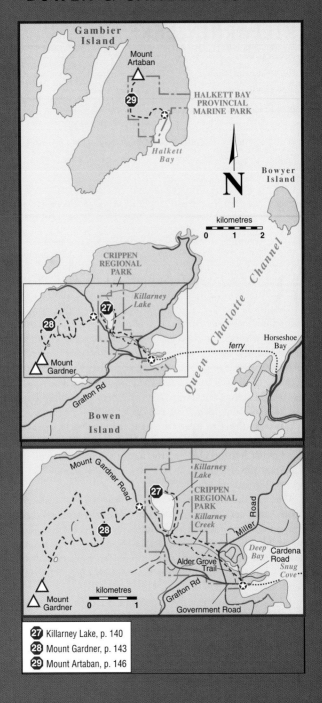

27 Killarney Lake, p. 140
28 Mount Gardner, p. 143
29 Mount Artaban, p. 146

27 KILLARNEY LAKE

Distance: 9 km	Rating: Easy
Elevation gain: Minimal	Season: Year-round
High point: 25 m	Topographical map:
Time needed: 2–4 hours	North Vancouver 92G/6
	Trail map: Page 139

Note: Dogs must be leashed. Wear footwear appropriate for muddy trails.

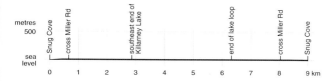

BOWEN ISLAND SEEMS TO BE FOREVER attracting visitors. In 1791, the Spanish explorer José María Narváez sailed into Howe Sound, spotted Bowen and named it Isla de Apodaca. A year later, Captain George Vancouver stopped in the area long enough to make a note in his journal of 'a number of Islands some of them pretty large & all coverd with Pines.' One of them, of course, was Bowen.

Although Bowen Island is just 15 kilometres from downtown Vancouver and a 20-minute ferry ride from Horseshoe Bay, one has the feeling of getting away from it all.

The first thing to leave behind is the car—at Horseshoe Bay. Or better yet, take the West Vancouver blue buses' scenic route along Marine Drive to the ferry terminal. (For sailing times and fares, contact BC Ferries at 1-888-223-3779 or www.bcferries.com.)

Once at the Snug Cove terminal, head up Government Road. Cafes and stores line the left side of the road, in case you want to start your day with coffee, breakfast or lunch. But the walking portion of this program begins across the street, near the old Union Steamship Company Store, which is now home to the post office and the Greater Vancouver Regional District (GVRD) offices.

About 100 metres east of the old store is a green and yellow GVRD Parks sign pointing the way to Killarney Lake. Head into the forest to the Bowen Memorial Garden for a short stroll through the garden area—in spring and summer there are lovely blooms; in fall and winter, there are good views of Deep Bay.

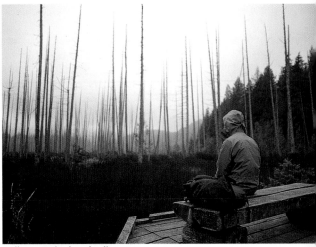

Killarney Lake, boardwalk section.

At the garden, head left along a trail that, in autumn, is carpeted with leaves fallen from the broadleaf maple and alder trees overhead. Soon, the trail forks. Both routes rejoin farther ahead, but take the right trail, because it's farther from the road and closer to the water.

Just after the trails meet, you'll hear the sound of the tumbling waters of Killarney Creek and the tiny Bridal Veil Falls, often swollen by rain. A side-trail leads down to concrete fish ladders, which help salmon head lakewards.

Before non-Native people came to BC, Bowen Island was a hunting and fishing ground for the Squamish people and home to villages such as Qwel-hoom, Naych-Chail-Kun and Kwumch-Nam. It was also designated as a neutral meeting place for feuding tribes, and it served as an overnight respite for other Natives travelling up or down the coast.

When you've soaked up enough creek ambiance, rejoin the main trail and follow it to Miller Road. Cross the road and head right (north) for about 200 metres, to the sign noting the continuation of the Killarney Lake Trail.

The way here can be muddy, especially if it's been raining. After about 500 metres of walking through the open alder forest, the trail forks. Both routes meet at the lake, but do both and take the left fork in and the right on the way out.

Once at the lake, head left along the road and look for the little dam, which was built in the 1920s to ensure a constant supply of drinking water for the island. The lake is no longer used for water supply, but is part of Crippen Regional Park

Bowen Island is still a cozy retreat and the perfect place to go for a walk through canopies of maple and cedar, along creek and lakeshore.

and home to herons, ducks and kingfishers.

Although you may have the fortune to espy a deer or two, the wildlife of Bowen Island is nothing like it used to be. After arriving in the 1870s, the first settlers poisoned all the wolves—a dark chapter for a gem of an island.

Just to the left of the dam, look for the trail heading towards shore and follow it. It is a loop that wraps around the lake, through groves of cedar and spruce, with occasional side-trails that feature clear views of the lake. The way is mostly level, but can be muddy and slippery—especially on the wooden bridges and boardwalk at the north end of the lake, so watch your footing.

Much of the 240-hectare Crippen Park was once an island resort operated by the Union Steamship Company. During the 1920s and '30s, the grounds were home to 180 cottages, six picnic areas, an 800-person dance pavilion and a bandshell for vaudeville shows. The resort faltered in the 1940s, but a few remnants of that golden era still remain.

Eventually, the trail circles completely around the lake and returns to the dirt road where you first emerged. Turn left and uphill for a bit, to the green and yellow sign that points the way back to Snug Cove. Then simply retrace your relaxed steps.

Leave enough time to snoop around the shops or indulge in an aprés-walk snack. The Snug on Bowen serves great baked goods and coffee. And Doc Morgan's has a pub upstairs serving pub fare, including Bowen Island ale from the local microbrewery.

MOUNT GARDNER

Distance: 10 km

Elevation gain: 500 m

High point: 720 metres

Time needed: 6 hours

Rating: Moderate

Season: Year-round

Topographical map:
North Vancouver 92G/6

Trail map: Page 139

Note: Distance given is from trailhead—3 km from ferry dock.
Bringing a bicycle is recommended.

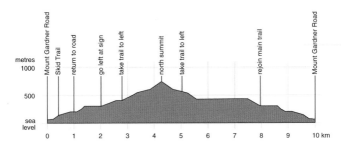

metres
1000

500

sea
level

0   1   2   3   4   5   6   7   8   9   10 km

Y OU WON'T HAVE TO LIFT A QUADRICEP FOR
the first view on this outing to Mount Gardner. All
you need to do is hop the ferry from Horseshoe Bay in
West Vancouver to Snug Cove on Bowen Island. For sailing
times and fares, contact BC Ferries at 1-888-223-3779 or
www.bcferries.com.

It's best to leave the car behind, but take a bicycle along for
the 3-kilometre journey to the trailhead. (That way, you don't
have to walk an extra 6 kilometres.)

After disembarking at Snug Cove, cycle to the first road on
the right: Cardena Drive. Turn right, and within 150 metres,
look left for the Alder Grove Trail heading into Crippen
Regional Park.

Fifteen minutes of cycling through groves of a mixed forest
of coniferous and deciduous trees brings you to Killarney Lake
and Magee Road. Go left to Mount Gardner Road, then bear
right, up a slightly killer hill. To take your mind off the huffing
and puffing, check the utility poles for identifying numbers.
When you spot pole number 490, look across the road for
the beginning of your mountain journey. The dirt and rock
roadway climbs steeply uphill for about 500 metres. If you can
ride your bike up, great. If you can't, walk your bike to the
gate, knowing that you're in good company.

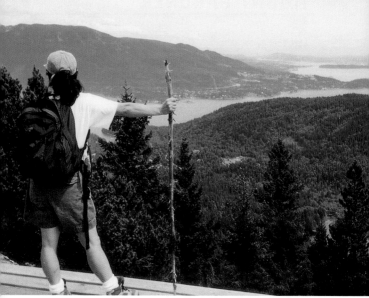

View from the top of Mount Gardner.

After locking your bike up and swigging a drink of water, it's time to hike. About 200 metres up the road, look to the left for the beginning of the Skid Trail, identified at first by pink ribbons tied to a tree, then orange markers and, farther, a sign.

The sign that tells you who to thank for this trip—the North Shore Hikers, who maintain the trail. Eventually, the Skid Trail rejoins the main road.

Head up the bumpy, grindy logging road to a fork in the road. Take the left tine as indicated by a handcrafted sign 'Mt. Gardner. Now comes the steep part' (hikers' humour). Eventually, you'll come to a microwave tower and a hut bearing a 'High Voltage' sign. Here, the logging road effectively ends, so follow the taped trail into the trees. After about 50 metres, the trail makes a sharp left up a wooded slope. Climb through this rather magical portion of baby trees, following the square orange markers.

The trail soon comes to a pond among the trees, which at certain times of year more resembles a bog. In summer, it's perfect breeding terrain for mosquitoes, so come equipped with bug spray. As you pass the pond and a little bridge, take note of where the Handloggers' Trail heads downhill to the right. On the way back from the summit, this will be the route down. For now, continue up a hillside, following the orange squares.

After 20 minutes of steady uphill, the trail emerges onto open rocky bluffs with views of Keats and Gambier islands and, farther beyond, the Sechelt Peninsula.

With its stellar views, the bluffs are a good place for a break. When you're ready, continue upwards to reach the north summit of Gardner. (The trail forks, but both lead to the north summit. The left fork is a bit more direct and thus a bit steeper.) From here, the views are 360°. Although the south summit is actually higher than this point, there are no views because of the lay of the land.

While you munch your lunch, think how different things might look if developers had gone ahead in the late 1960s with plans to transform Gardner into a ski hill as part of a $6-million overall plan that also called for an 18-hole golf course, shopping centre, service station and 1000 homes—each 100-unit 'colony' with its own swimming pool.

When you've finished lunching and resting and are ready for the trip back, simply retrace your steps to the pond. Then bear left onto the Handloggers' Trail. Travel steeply downhill for about 20 to 30 minutes, availing yourself of trees and branches along the way for stability.

For the next 45 minutes, traipse through mixed forest, dappled with sunlight and filled with bird song. As the trail descends, look for short side-trails, which lead to viewpoints on the rocky bluffs just beyond the shrubs and saplings.

The first viewpoint is on the left, with a great view of Killarney Lake below, Snug Cove and West Vancouver nearby and, way in the distance, a rarely seen aspect of downtown Vancouver. The second viewpoint is a little lower down, on the right. It makes for a good rest-break before the final descent.

Soon, the trail meets the main road again. Head down about 200 metres to find the start of the Skid Trail, and follow it back to the start and to your bike. Enjoy the ride down.

29 MOUNT ARTABAN

Distance: 10 km	Rating: Moderate
Elevation gain: 610 m	Season: Year-round
High point: 610 m	Topographical map:
Time needed: 6 hours	North Vancouver 92G/6
	Trail map: Page 139

Note: Gambier Island is accessible only by boat. Bring drinking water. None is available at Halkett Bay or on the trail.

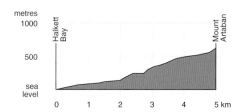

WHEN MOST FOLKS THINK OF ISLANDS, they think of water-related activities such as kayaking, canoeing and sailing. But many of BC's islands are great hiking destinations as well.

On Bowen Island, there's Mount Gardner; on Saltspring Island, there's Ruckle Park; on Mayne Island, there's Mount Parke. All of these islands are served by BC Ferries, and all are good for dayhikes if you're spending some of your summer in the Strait of Georgia.

Close to Vancouver, there's another great hike accessible only by water—Mount Artaban on Gambier Island. Since BC Ferries does not send any of its fleet there, you'll need access to a boat to get there. I paddled to Gambier, by kayak, from Lions Bay. Go this route and you're in for a long day—or an overnight camping stay. Crossing times depend on weather and water conditions. (Under ideal conditions, I took 90 minutes to cover the 10 kilometres from Lions Bay to Halkett Bay Provincial Marine Park.)

Allow six hours for the hike alone. And be sure to bring a minimum of 2 litres drinking water per person—none is available at the bay or on the trail.

Enter Halkett Bay Provincial Marine Park by boat and anchor or beach your craft. Then from the dock at the bay's head, follow the trail into the woods, watching for the pink tape and orange diamond-shaped markers that indicate the way. At first, the trail wanders along a small stream, under a canopy

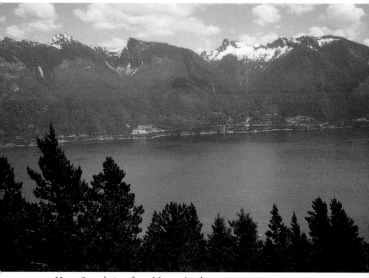

Howe Sound view from Mount Artaban.

of mixed forest—alder and maple, cedar and fir, breaking occasionally into a small sunlit grove of giant purply-pink foxgloves.

After about 20 minutes of level ground, the trail rises for a few minutes of heavy breathing, then levels again. Not much farther is a handprinted sign noting the 1-kilometre mark, and not much farther again, an intersection. The trail to the left leads to Camp Fircom, run by the United Church of Canada.

We, however, will go right and follow the trail as it winds upward through an area choked with wood debris. As you duck under and wander around the fallen branches and trunks, don't forget to take in the one benefit of so many downed trees—the first glimpse of the peaks across Howe Sound. The trail levels and comes to another intersection, this time with the Cross Trail, which, not surprisingly, leads left to the cross perched on a rocky ridge above Camp Fircom.

But we will again go right. Follow the orange diamonds and tape into a clearcut area, now in the initial stages of growing back—thus full of foxgloves, giant ferns and other meadow foliage. Keep your eyes on the markers as you wade through the 2-metre-high fern forest and whack your way to the rocky benchland a couple of hundred metres distant.

From here, the trail traverses along the upper margins of the cut—you can see it, and some peeks of Bowen, Keats and Pasley islands, on your left. Here, where the forest is more

On top of Mount Artaban you'll find the splintered remnants of an old Forest Service lookout, 360° views of Howe Sound and clouds of swallowtail butterflies.

open, the scents of resin, wood and needles fill the air. Each step seems to release a fresh fragrant cloud, tempting you to breathe in just a bit deeper.

After an easy hour or so on the trail is a handprinted 2-kilometre sign, and a few minutes farther, another intersection. Here, go in the direction pointed out by the wooden sign—right and up.

The mountain proper lies ahead; no more gentle sloping followed by level ground. From now on, it's a steady slog to the top. For the first 40 to 50 minutes, the trail climbs alongside a gully, then, just where a massive tree has fallen across the gully, at the foot of a burned-out cedar snag, the trail bears right and uphill again.

From here it's a 20- to 25-minute grunt up sometimes steep, rocky terrain. Then finally, the summit. The views from Artaban are really one of a kind. From here, the entire mountain ridge that makes up the Howe Sound Crest lies before as nowhere else. On the far right, above Horseshoe Bay, is Black Mountain; moving north is Mount Strachan, St. Mark's Summit, Unnecessary Mountain and the Lions (only the West Lion is visible from here), then Harvey, Brunswick and Hat mountains and finally, Deeks Peak.

To the north, peaks in the Tantalus Range and in Garibaldi Provincial Park are visible, including a distant view of Black Tusk. To the west are some of the summits in the newly created Tetrahedron Wilderness Area. To the south are views of Bowen Island, Greater Vancouver and the San Juan Islands in the US.

They're the same sights that bedazzled Captain George Vancouver and his naturalist Archibald Menzies in 1792, when they first sailed into Howe Sound to find 'stupendous snowy mountains rising almost perpendicular from the Water's edge.'

After all the effort spent to get to the top, take an hour or so and enjoy these long-appreciated views. Then, head back down the trail the way you came.

HOWE SOUND

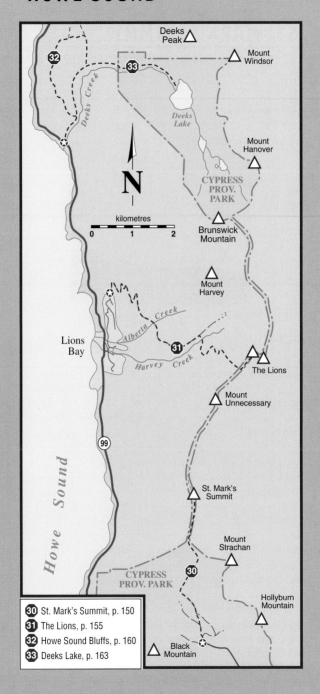

Deeks Peak

32

33

Mount Windsor

Deeks Creek

Deeks Lake

N

Mount Hanover

CYPRESS PROV. PARK

kilometres
0   1   2

Brunswick Mountain

Mount Harvey

Alberta Creek

Lions Bay

31

Harvey Creek

The Lions

Mount Unnecessary

99

St. Mark's Summit

Mount Strachan

Howe Sound

Hollyburn Mountain

30

CYPRESS PROV. PARK

Black Mountain

30 ST. MARK'S SUMMIT

Distance: 11 km	Rating: Moderate
Elevation gain: 460 m	Season: July to October
High point: 1335 m	Topographical map:
Time needed: 5 hours	North Vancouver 92G/6
	Trail map: Page 149

Note: Dogs must be leashed.

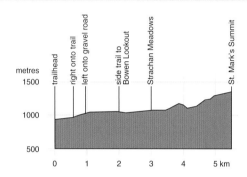

THE HOWE SOUND CREST TRAIL STRETCHES for 30 kilometres from Cypress Bowl through subalpine meadows, lakes and forested groves over ridges and mountains to emerge on Highway 99 just south of Porteau Cove.

It's more than a little long for a dayhike, but the section that traipses happily to St. Mark's Summit will give a good sense of the nature of the Howe Sound Crest Trail and, perhaps, inspiration for a future backpack adventure.

To get to the trailhead, follow the Upper Levels Highway to West Vancouver and take exit #8 to Cypress Provincial Park. Follow the Cypress Parkway up to the uppermost parking lot.

At the BC Parks signboard, pick up a park brochure/map and follow the path north towards the chairlift. Soon, you'll pass signs that note the paths heading left to Yew Lake, a short, sweet destination filled with natural wonders and encircled by a wheelchair-accessible trail.

Continue straight through, following the signs that point to the Howe Sound Crest Trail. At first, you traipse along a dusty, rocky road, then briefly into the trees, then back to the dusty, rocky road. A few minutes later the road dwindles to an end right where the BC Parks sign indicates that you are entering a wilderness area.

Sunshine Coast, from top of St. Mark's Summit.

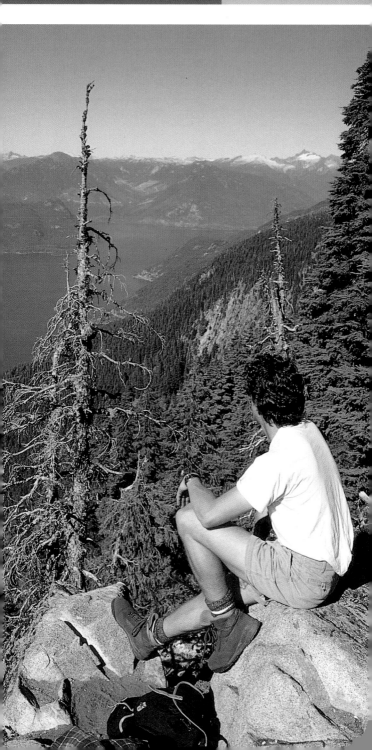

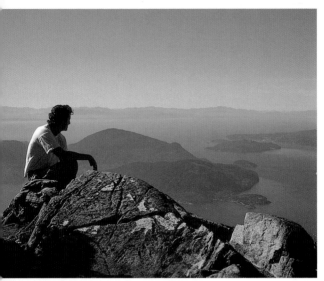

View of Bowen and Vancouver islands.

Follow the trail as it skirts the lower slopes of Mount Strachan, through cool, quiet, untouched forests. Before logging and ski resorts scarred the bowl area, the whole valley looked like this.

Before Cypress was set aside as a provincial park, various private companies logged in the area. In the late 1930s, the Los Angeles-based Heaps Timber Company logged more than 40 hectares on Hollyburn and in the Cypress Valley, prompting controversy and political negotiations. As a result, Cypress Bowl was set aside in 1944 as a park reserve.

Then in 1966, Mountain Timbers Ltd. was hired to clear an area slated for ski resort development that featured a 7000-house subdivision and parking space for 5000 cars. In less than two years, the company logged more than 10 million board feet of timber from Mount Strachan's lower slopes.

A couple of years ago, more trees came down for expansion of the downhill ski facilities. And although that is hardly cause for celebration, it is much less than was first proposed. The new company that operates the commercial facilities has also indicated that it no longer wants to build a restaurant on top of Mount Strachan, saving much old-growth and wildlife habitat.

It's something to contemplate as you continue to a junction with a short side-trail to Bowen Lookout—worth a look for the few minutes it takes. Just a few steps farther is the Lions View Lookout on the right. Again, it's worth a look.

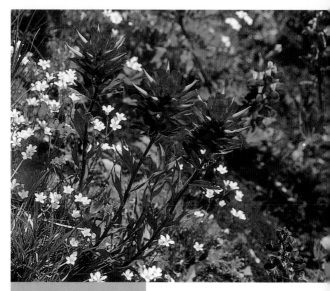

In summer, wildflowers such as arctic lupine, Sitka valerian and Indian paint-brush abound. In the fall, the rustic red, orange and yellow foliage adds colour and a particular autumn scent to the scene.

Once back on the main trail, continue along as the trail dips to cross Monti-zambert Creek then winds upwards into the beauty of Strachan Meadows.

Feel free to dawdle, even to rest. Not because you're tired, just because you want to enjoy the meadows and the mountains. From here, the trail climbs upward for the next 15 to 20 minutes, zigging and zagging until it reaches the height of one ridge at 1180 metres. On the left are views of Howe Sound. On the right is a small meadow.

Continue straight to another summit, then descend into a muddy bit. Then it's up again through another series of switchbacks. At times, the trail is a tangle of tree roots. Watch your footing, because these roots can make even the most nimble hiker look like he's doing a Jerry Lewis impression.

Eventually, you'll reach the top of the rise and wander through the first subalpine meadows of St. Mark's. Side-trails lead to viewpoints over Howe Sound, but you're not quite there yet. Continue a bit farther through the meadows, making sure to stay on the trail. And clamber across the rocky knolls. The gray jays and the views will tell you when you've arrived.

Here, at the summit of St. Mark's, you are 1335 metres directly above sea level. Looking west, you can see all the way from the islands of Howe Sound to the glaciers of the Tantalus Range. On a clear day, the peaks of various Gulf Islands and even Vancouver Island can be seen. Looking down the precipitous slopes to Highway 99, the cars look like tiny scuttling mice.

It is a stunning view. And if you have the fortune to be there at a time when no one else is about, it seems as close to paradise as one can come sitting on a rocky outcrop.

Speaking of heavenly matters, you might be interested to know that St. Mark is the patron of cattle breeders, Venice, notaries and glaziers. But I think the name of the summit may have come from someone who'd forgotten bug spray. Mark, you see, is also the saint invoked against fly bites.

Kick back, eat lunch and absorb all the sights, sounds and smells. Bring some unsalted sunflower seeds for the gray jays, and the northwestern chipmunks if they ever stop chattering and scampering. Listen for the throaty trills of a spruce grouse tucked in the underbrush. Then, when you can bear it, retrace your steps to the parking area.

THE LIONS

Distance: Up to 16 km	Season: July to October
Elevation gain: 1300 m	Topographical map:
High point: 1575 m	North Vancouver 92G/6
Time needed: Up to 7 hours	Trail map: Page 149
Rating: Strenuous	

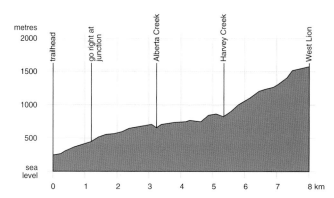

THE HIKE TO THE MOST RECOGNIZABLE geographical landmark in the Lower Mainland is a popular one. But it is not by any means easy. Although our route covers the entire trip to the base of the West Lion, it's also possible to make a somewhat shorter trip that gives equally terrific views.

To get to the trailhead, head north on Highway 99 and take the Lions Bay turnoff onto Oceanview Road. Turn left at Cross Creek Road and cross Harvey Creek, then go right on Centre Road. At Bayview Road, go left to Mountain Drive, then left again. At Sunset make a final left. Parking spaces at the end of the road are few, so go early or be prepared to park 1 kilometre down the road at Lions Bay School and to add another 30 to 45 minutes to your outing.

Pass around the yellow gate and follow a wide dirt road through a forest, which was logged not all that long ago. Still, sizable cedars and moss-covered broadleaf maples are growing back. Where the road curves, the ascent changes from gradual uphill to committed grunt.

The sound of Magnesia Creek burbles happily below and soon after, the road reaches a junction with a view of Mount Harvey. Go right. (The road straight ahead leads to Mount Brunswick.) The familiar orange marker about 25 metres up the road lets you know you're going the right way.

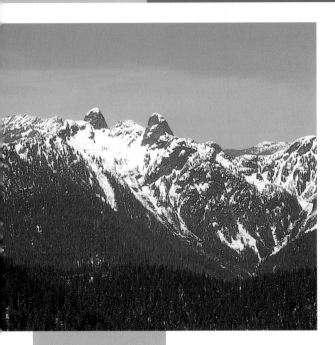

Twenty to 25 minutes of constant uphill grinding later, the road meets another junction. Again, go right, this time following an arrow of stones that has been cleverly built in the middle of the path. (Left goes to Mount Brunswick.) Soon after, the road grade mercifully eases from unrelenting to steady and, eventually, to level.

The trail is an old skid road, as evidenced from the occasional logging remnant—lengths of thick rusted wire cable and big stumps. As the path continues, the roar of Highway 99 traffic seeps through the second-growth trees along the trail. Not much further, the forest opens to reveal a view of Mount Unnecessary to the right and the ridge below the West Lion directly ahead. Where the trail crosses rockfall is the first really good view—southwest to Bowyer,

Bowen and Passage islands, Horseshoe Bay, and in the distance, some of the Gulf and San Juan islands.

Just beyond, big trees begin to appear on the steeper downslope side of the trail: stately Douglas firs, towering hemlock and spruce. A few minutes farther, the road narrows and crosses Alberta Creek, which cascades down a rock bluff in a lacy waterfall. A short uphill section features another point with views of Mount Artaban on Gambier Island (see page 146) and the Sunshine Coast.

About 15 minutes later, the trail splits. Go right and downslope toward Harvey Creek, following the pink tape. (Left goes to Harvey Creek Meadows.) Just before the creek is a sign noting the people responsible for maintaining the trail: the BC Mountaineering Club. Unfortunately, the sign does not mention the man almost solely responsible for building the trail in the first place: the late Paul Binkert. Until Binkert flagged and cleared the trail in 1971, putting in stairs and other improvements along the way, people used to make a nine-hour return hike to the Lions via Mount Unnecessary.

Cross the creek carefully—there's no bridge. If you haven't taken a water break already, do it here. The next section is a long, steady grunt. Follow the markers and the trail uphill through lush rainforest. Underfoot are branchlets of cedar and needles of hemlock and fir. Big western red cedar and Douglas fir abound on the boulder-strewn way. From here on, the hiking is superb, but you'll work for it.

The trail wriggles back and forth at first, like a snake trying to set itself free. Just keep eyeballing the orange and silver markers to stay on track. After 30 to 40 minutes of steady ascent through sweetly scented forest, across ancient boulder fields, and over and around blowdown, the trail arrives to a splendid viewpoint of Howe Sound.

From here, the trees seem to get bigger, thicker, more awesome, but maybe it's the effect of endless switchbacks up and across the final steep slope. Where blue sky begins to peek teasingly through the tree tops, the slope steepens just a bit more making for a scramble up tangles of exposed tree roots and mud. Thirty to 40 minutes after the viewpoint, the trail levels then makes a final short spurt to the ridge and bam! The West Lion stands before you.

This spot can be your lunch stop and turnaround point, but there is an even more stunning vantage point just five to 10 minutes farther up the trail among the meadows with views of Howe Sound and beyond, in addition to the West Lion.

For hikers who have more energy, it's possible to continue up, up, up the meadows and boulders to a gully that eventually

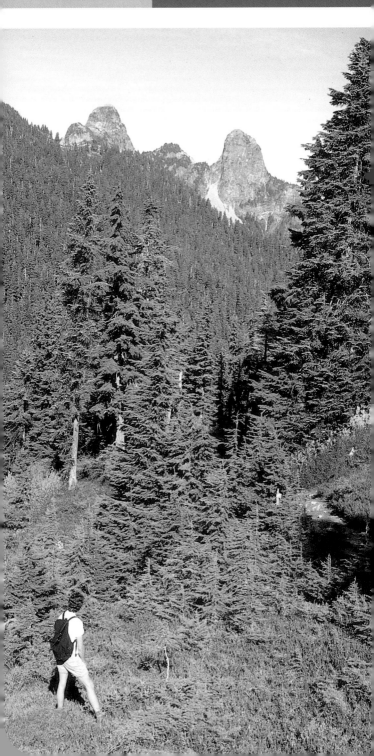

leads to a higher ridge with a view of the East Lion and points east. The Lions Trail technically ends just above the saddle to the West Lion. And although you may see people scrambling up or down the peak, remember that it is not a hike. It is steep and exposed and best left to those with rock-climbing expertise. Each year, people fall from the West Lion. The lucky are only injured, but there have been several fatalities.

Wherever the summit of your day's hike is, take a moment to remember the story of The Two Sisters, as told by Chief Joe Capilano to Pauline Johnson, and related in her book *Legends of Vancouver*.

Many thousands of years ago, Johnson tells us, a great chief had two daughters who both came of age the same spring. Their father prepared to make a feast in celebration and the people looked forward to many days of rejoicing, dancing and eating.

There was, however, a shadow cast on the festivities. The chief had been warring with peoples who lived near Prince Rupert. War parties paddled the coast, their songs breaking the night's silence, stirring more hatred, vengeance and strife. But the chief, having won every encounter, turned away from battle to feast in his daughters' honour.

A week before the appointed feast day, the daughters asked their father to grant them a favour. 'The favour is yours before you ask it,' the chief replied. So they asked him to invite his enemies to the feast. The chief, although surprised, honoured his daughters' wish and sent his men to welcome the enemy. The northern peoples emptied the war canoes of their weapons and filled them instead with game and fish, beads and baskets, carved ladles and woven blankets, then with the women and children of the village, the warriors paddled south.

At the feast, the two peoples laid aside their hostilities and forged an alliance. In recognition of their selfless deed, the Sagalie Tyee (God) made the two young maidens immortal.

'In the cup of his hands,' related Chief Capilano, 'he lifted the chief's two daughters and set them forever in a high place.'

After paying your respects to The Sisters, retrace your steps to the trailhead.

The Lions as seen from Strachan Meadows.

32 HOWE SOUND BLUFFS

Distance: 10 km

Elevation gain: 400 m

High point: 465 m

Time needed: 5 hours

Rating: Moderate

Season: May to October

Topographical map:
Squamish 92G/11

Trail map: Page 149

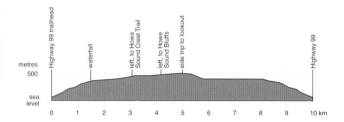

BIG VIEWS, BIG TREES AND A BOG. THIS HIKE has them all. The trails that meander through the bluffs area are wonderful studies in contrast. Some trails thread through a damp forest fecund with Sitka spruce and Douglas fir, others wind around rocky outcrops and stunted scrub pine.

The only caution on this hike is that with so many trails—and some overgrowth—things can get confusing. There is no really good map of the area, but the signs and markers should keep you on the right track.

To get to the trailhead, follow Highway 99 past Lions Bay. About 11 kilometres past Lions Bay, look for a big pullout on the west side of the highway. If there is no oncoming traffic, you can pull in. If not—and there is also no traffic behind you—you can wait. Otherwise, go 200 metres farther and use the turnaround on your side of the road.

The trickiest part of the trip may be recrossing the road on foot to the trailhead sign. Vehicle traffic is very fast here, so be very, very careful.

From the sign, follow the trail up and along the edges of Kallahne Creek. In summer, it's nice and cool here and there's even a waterfall to distract you on the steady uphill. After 20 minutes of hiking, the trail levels and brings you to your first views of the day. A few minutes farther are even more views from atop a rocky outcrop. It's a good stop for a water break.

Then follow the trail into the forest and up, up, up. About 20 minutes farther, the trail meets an old road. Go right. Not much farther, you might notice a small sign on an alder tree: "28.5 km." No, you haven't gone that far already. It's

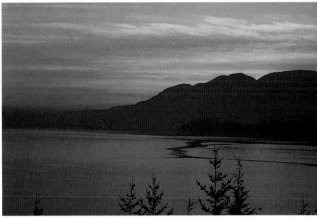

Setting sun over Howe Sound.

in reference to the Howe Sound Crest Trail and how far you would have come had you started at the southern trailhead in Cypress Provincial Park.

Continue up the old road, checking out the wildflowers, forest and forest critters (mostly squirrels and birds) on the way. About 45 minutes of hiking brings you to a junction. Left goes to Deeks Lake (see page 163), but we'll go right to the bluffs.

Within 10 minutes walking, the trail comes to a boggy area. Look on the right hand (south) side of the bog for a trail. It's a bit indistinct at first, but as you follow it along the edge of the bog, the path opens up. Be sure to check out the bog as well. There are all kinds of neat little plants here, including the tiny round-leaved sundew (*Drosera rotundifolia*), an insectivorous plant that snares mosquitoes, gnats and midges with its sticky tentacles and gobbles them up.

Pass the side-trail on the left (it ends at a pond) and climb upward until you reach a junction. (You can't miss it; it's right where a small pine tree sits in the middle of the trail.)

Go right. And, a few metres farther, right again. Scramble up the trail to reach the high point — 465 metres — and absolutely stunning views. It's the perfect place to have lunch.

Similar views were mentioned by one of the first travellers to the area—Archibald Menzies, the naturalist on board the *Discovery*, Captain George Vancouver's ship. In his 1792 journal, Menzies wrote of sailing from Burrard Inlet into Howe Sound: "We soon after enterd an Arm leading to the Northward about a mile & a quarter wide & formed on both sides by ridges of stupendous snowy mountains rising almost perpendicular from the Water's edge."

From your perch, Anvil and Gambier islands part the waters immediately below, and the peaks of the Sunshine Coast—Mount Elphinstone, Panther and Tetrahedron Peaks—form a formidable backdrop.

When you're ready, scramble back down to the main trail. You could call it a day and retrace your steps to the highway. But if you're up for more, go right. Fifteen to 20 minutes of walking brings you to a rocky bluff with more great views. Continue on the trail for another 10 minutes or so.

The next part may be tricky, so pay attention. An old cat-track used to branch left and connect to the Deeks Lake trail. These days, it's pretty much grown over with alder and brush. But you never know, someone may decide to clear it out.

Your best bet is to stay with the orange markers and signs that point towards the bluffs. That will get you to the main trail that traverses a long undulating ridge with sections of dry forest interspersed with viewpoints—each one just a bit different than the one before.

You also have the option of doing a side loop into the forest east of the ridge. It will add to your overall distance and elevation gain, but there are some spots that make it worth the trip. Small groves of big old Douglas fir and Sitka spruce still stand, and sections of blowdown can leave you in awe of the power of wind. The cool waters of Deeks Creek can provide some temperature relief.

There are two points where side-trails split off. If you take the first, you can drop down into the forest and check things out. At the next junction, you'd then go right and follow the forest trail south to another junction. Hang a right and go back up to the top of the bluffs. Then go right and head northward on the bluffs trail to start the return trip.

The bluffs trail does continue south to emerge onto the highway near Deeks Creek, but it ends about five kilometres south of where you left your vehicle.

DEEKS LAKE

Distance: 13 km	Season: July to October
Elevation gain: 980 m	Topographical map:
High point: 1030 m	Squamish 92G/11
Time needed: 7 hours	Trail map: Page 149
Rating: Strenuous	

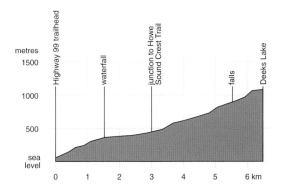

IT'S A LONG, FULL DAY OF HIKING, BUT WHEN such a day starts with views of Howe Sound, progresses through big trees and alongside waterfalls, and arrives at a beautiful alpine lake, who's going to complain? Just allow for a long break at the top, whether it's to explore the lakeshore, take a dip in the chilly waters or get in some quality catnapping.

To get to the trailhead, head up Highway 99 towards Lions Bay. Then start checking the names of the creeks. Six kilometres past Lions Bay, just after Loggers Creek, is Deeks Creek. Park in the big pullout on the west side of the highway before Deeks Creek. Or go a few kilometres past the creek, turn around and drive back to the smaller pullout just opposite Deeks. Either option is safer than turning left across the highway on a blind corner.

(It's also possible to begin the hike about 5 kilometres farther north on Highway 99 at the northern end of the Howe Sound Crest Trail. It's about the same distance, but not as scenic a beginning as the creekside access.)

Be very careful crossing the highway on foot to the trailhead. Then look for the orange squares that mark the old trail on the left bank of Deeks Creek.

The first 15 to 20 minutes is a steep hands-and-feet scramble, often made slippery by recent rainfall. But there are two viewpoints along the way, the first looking out over

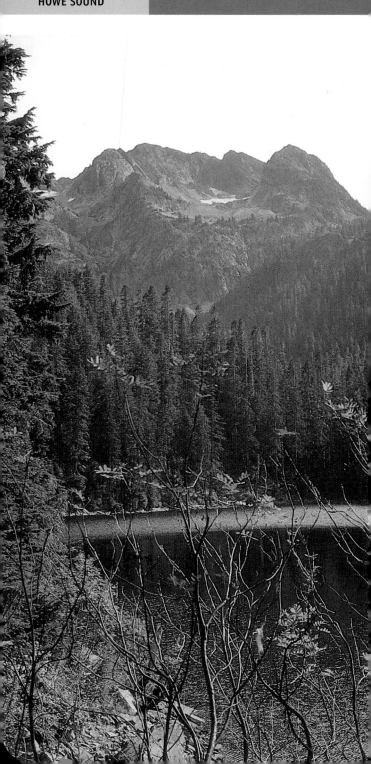

Howe Sound and Deeks Creek below, and the second an even more stunning vista of the islands, ocean and mountain slopes that make the Sound what it is.

Soon, the trail levels and enters the forest. After 20 to 30 minutes, the creek is once again visible from the trail. Make a short detour right to see a beautiful little waterfall.

A few steps farther brings you to the northern shore, which is often still snow-covered through July, and a full view of all its exquisite nature: deep blue waters, quiet lakeside marsh and the dramatically steep slopes all around.

For the next 45 minutes or so, as the trail wanders through a cathedral of Douglas fir and Sitka spruce. Many of BC's Native Peoples believed that the sharp needles of the Sitka spruce gave it powers against evil thoughts. Its boughs were used by the Ditidaht and Nuu-chah-nulth peoples in winter dance ceremonies. Spruce pitch was used as a medicine for burns, colds and toothaches among other ailments.

A bit farther along the trail is a section of blowdown where some of the forest giants have fallen victim to high winds. Stay with the orange markers to a white 'shortcut' sign, and follow its direction through a grove of alders to emerge onto a cat-track, left behind by old logging operations.

Soon, you're at a trail junction. Go right to follow the signs and orange metal markers towards Deeks Lake. (Left is the Howe Sound Crest Trail heading to Highway 99 and the turning point for the Howe Sound Bluffs Trail, described on page 160.)

The path heads uphill, old roads and alternate trails deviating to its right and left. (One old road heads to the dilapidated remnants of an old homestead before being washed out by the creek a few steps farther.) The next section of the trail can be a bit confusing, because a bank over which the original route clambered has slid. Although some people still clamber up the slump to gain the original route into the trees above, it's also possible to stay uphill on an alternate trail, marked by red tape and orange markers, which rejoins the main trail about 1.5 kilometres distant. (That's 20 to 30 minutes later, depending on your pace.)

Whichever route you choose, just be sure to continue following those orange metal markers—the hiker's equivalent of a directional security blanket. The trail travels steadily upward, crossing the occasional seasonal creek until 15 minutes or so

Mount Brunswick and Deeks Lake.

later you reach the tumbling majesty of Phi Alpha Falls. Take a moment to soak up some of the ambiance, take a water break and rest your feet. There's still a stiffish kilometre to climb.

Then put one foot in front of the other and continue trudging up the trail, across another couple of seasonal creeks, and up a hands-and-feet scramble through a damp forested section to emerge to more level ground with a view down the creek canyon.

Stay with the orange markers for another 10 to 15 minutes upward until finally you hit level ground and get the first glimpse of Deeks Lake. The slopes to the north belong to Deeks Peak, the slope to the east to Mount Windsor, and the slopes to the southwest to a nameless 1470-metre bump.

It's hard to imagine that Deeks Lake hasn't always been here. But in fact, it's only about 85 years old. A wooden dam built about 1910 stopped the flow of Deeks Creek to create the lake and provide water for the Deeks Sand and Gravel Company below.

The lake, the creek and the peak above are all named for the owner of the company, John Deeks, who first began working the slopes for sand and gravel in 1908.

The Howe Sound Crest Trail continues around the west shore of the lake, then climbs higher to a lake sometimes known as Upper Deeks, other times as Hanover, and on and on for another 23 or so kilometres to emerge at Cypress Bowl. That's a trip best saved for a future long weekend of backpacking. So find a spot at lakeside and enjoy, before retracing your steps to the parking area on Highway 99.

SQUAMISH AREA

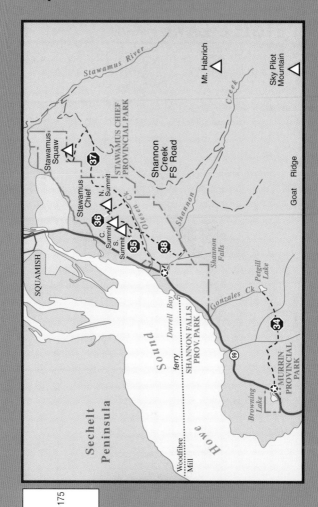

Stawamus River

Mt. Habrich

Sky Pilot Mountain

Stawamus Squaw

STAWAMUS CHIEF PROVINCIAL PARK

Shannon Creek FS Road

Creek

Goat Ridge

Stawamus Chief

N. Summit

C. Summit

S. Summit

Oleson Ck

Shannon

SQUAMISH

Shannon Falls

Petgill Lake

Darrell Bay

Gonzales Ck

ferry

SHANNON FALLS PROV. PARK

99

MURRIN PROVINCIAL PARK

Sound

Howe

Sechelt Peninsula

Woodfibre Mill

Browning Lake

N

kilometres
0   1   2

34 PETGILL LAKE

Distance: 12 km	Rating: Moderate
Elevation gain: 610 m	Season: March to October
High point: 760 m	Topographical map:
Time needed: 6 hours	Squamish 92G/11
	Trail map: Page 167

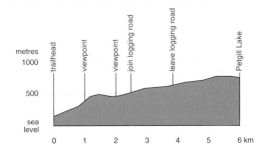

H OWE SOUND VIEWS AND TRANQUIL
forest line the way to tiny jewel-like Petgill Lake.
Although the sights may not rival those of the Chief
and Garibaldi Provincial Park farther north, the hike to Petgill
Lake is the perfect outing for an overcast day in spring or fall.
It can also be a good destination for a blazingly hot summer
day, but be warned that in clear weather it's much easier to see
the wide swathe of forest that has been recently mowed down
behind the lake.

To get to the trailhead, follow Highway 99 north to the
parking lot at Murrin Provincial Park, about 2 kilometres north
of Britannia Beach.

On foot, head north from the lot and across to the
highway's east side. About 500 metres farther is the start of
the trail proper. For the first few minutes the trail scrambles
upward among a tangle of rocks, roots and blowdown that
require some tricky moves and, at times, hands as well as feet.
Move slowly and carefully, being sure to follow the pink and
orange tapes.

Stay left where the trail forks (right is an access route for
rock-climbers). And follow the trail as it heads north along the
bluff ridge. Ten minutes farther, the trail comes to a trio of
hydro pylons and views open across to Mount Roderick and
other nameless peaks on the western Sechelt Peninsula.

Where a big hunk of granite outcrops onto the trail, stay
high and look for two orange diamonds adorning a stump.
(The lower trail again is access to a rock-climbing area.) A final

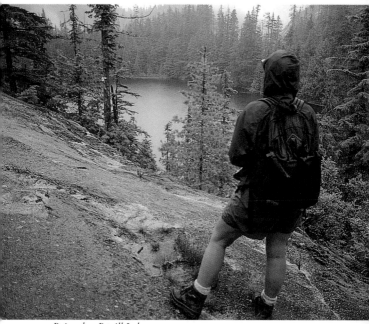

Rainy day, Petgill Lake.

scramble up and the trail enters a forest of stately Douglas fir, western hemlock and Sitka spruce.

A few minutes farther, where you near a deep damp gully, moisture-loving western red cedars make their appearance. Where a seasonal creek trickles through, the trail goes right to continue uphill. At the next bluff, follow the trail up and to the right.

Not much farther is a viewpoint featuring views of the waters of Howe Sound, the mountains across and the lights of Woodfibre Mill, with a small community of microwave transmitters perched on the opposite bluff.

Not all that long ago, before chemical plants and pulp mills called Howe Sound home, you might have seen a pod of killer whales gliding by. Gray whales once also frequented these waters, but that was even longer ago, before overhunting had decimated their population by the 1950s.

From here, the trail descends into another gully of cedars. One ancient snag is riddled with woodpecker holes. (I stopped counting at 100.) The most likely suspects are western pileated woodpeckers. These crow-sized birds also drill large oval- or rectangular-shaped holes for nesting. Once they've abandoned the sites, other animals such as squirrels and small owls move in.

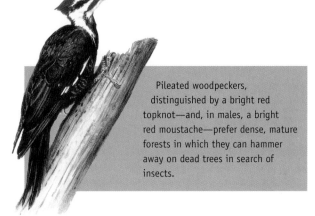

Pileated woodpeckers, distinguished by a bright red topknot—and, in males, a bright red moustache—prefer dense, mature forests in which they can hammer away on dead trees in search of insects.

Just beyond the woodpeckered tree is a short side-trail leading to another viewpoint, which looks north to the Stawamus Chief and the Squamish River estuary. A few minutes farther is the last lookout with even better views of the Chief and river.

From here, the trail descends to join an old logging road on which you'll bear right and uphill. Ten to 15 minutes farther, the old road crosses a nameless creek, and then a few minutes farther, recrosses it. Continue uphill and through a section that can be overgrown at times with roadside foliage.

After 10 minutes of pseudo-bushwhacking, where the old road is blocked and really overgrown, look for a marker on the left where the trail leads into the forest. Follow it up to a ridge top, which affords some glimpses of Howe Sound, then continue down into a marshy saddle.

From here, the trail goes on a 25- to 30-minute dipsy-doodle traverse dropping into a gully, up another ridge and through a moss-covered rock canyon. Soon, you'll have to ascend a bare rock outcrop, then drop through a narrow cleft in the granite into a deep dark gully.

As you ascend on the other side, a vast granite wall looms left of the rail. Dipsy-doodle for another 15 to 20 minutes to a trail junction. Continue straight. (Right is a route used by experienced backcountry hikers and climbers to Goat Ridge and Sky Pilot Mountain, some hours distant.)

Another 10 minutes on the trail brings you to Petgill Lake. On the best days, tendrils of mist swirl in and around the surrounding trees and cloak the logged-out area behind. The lake takes its name from two engineers at Britannia Mine—Peterson and Gillmore—who lived at the Mount

Sheer townsite and came upon this little lake while exploring their bigger neighbourhood. It soon became a popular picnic spot for families.

There are various vantage points on the trail encircling the lake from which to enjoy your own picnic and the views of Goat Ridge to the southeast.

Prospectors are believed to have been the first to climb the ridge, well before the beginning of the 20th century. Pre-World War I records indicate that claims were staked in a large area encompassing the ridge, Sky Pilot, Red Mountain and Mount Baldwin. Remember, it's quite near Brittania Beach, where copper was first discovered in 1888.

The Brittania Mine opened in 1905 and soon became the largest producer of copper in the British Empire. By the time the last shift at the mine punched the clock in 1979, the mine had produced 500,000 tonnes of copper, 122,000 tonnes of zinc, 15,000 tonnes of lead, 14 million grams of gold and 84 million grams of silver.

But the community paid a price for the natural riches: In 1915, an avalanche killed 58 people, and in 1921, a flood burst a dam in Britannia Creek, killing 37 residents. Subsequent floods in 1933 and in the 1960s resulted in a decision to breach the dams, high above in the creek's headwaters, which formerly held reservoirs for the mining operations.

When you've sated yourself with lakeside munching and musing, retrace your steps through the forest, past the viewpoints and down the rocky, rooty tangle at the beginning to Murrin Park.

35 STAWAMUS CHIEF: SOUTH SUMMIT

Distance: 7 km	Rating: Moderate
Elevation gain: 500 m	Season: March to November
High point: 600 m	Topographical map:
Time needed: 3–4 hours	Squamish 92G/11
	Trail map: Page 167

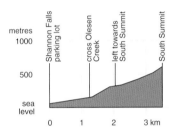

IF YOU'VE BEEN TO SQUAMISH, YOU'VE SEEN the Chief's looming granite profile. During the summer, its face is usually daubed with small blobs of colour—rock climbers taking the vertical route to the top.

What you can't see is a system of trails tucked in behind the granite massif for those folks who prefer a more gradual ascent, without ropes, without the dizzying intricacies of smearing, jamming and stemming one's way to the top.

Make no mistake though. The trails are also tremendously popular. Of the 50,000 people who hike the Chief each year, most go in the months of June, July, August and September. A sunny day is virtually a guarantee of a long conga line of people trudging to the top, some woefully ill-prepared in sandals or heels, carrying no water and whose regular physical exercise involves going from the couch to the fridge.

The hike to the South Summit is best done in spring or fall when it's not as busy, preferably on a cloudy or overcast day.

To get to the trailhead, follow Highway 99 north towards Squamish. One kilometre past Shannon Falls Provincial Park, turn right at the first Stawamus Chief Provincial Park entrance. Stay right on the road to the walk-in campground. Park in the areas designated for non-campers.

Head for the park sign on the left of the road, and follow the trail through the campground to the sound of Olesen Creek and the start of the Stawamus Chief Trail.

Scramble up a rock outcrop and start your steady diet of uphill. From here, it's straight up on stone steps and wooden stairs. In a few minutes, a side-trail branches right to Shannon Falls park. Take a breather and check out the views from the bridge. Then continue upward.

This part of the trail gets a lot of use and has had some badly needed repairs thanks to the Stawamus Chief (and Squaw) receiving long-awaited recognition in 1995 under BC's Protected Areas Strategy. Now, it's the Stawamus Chief Provincial Park.

At the first fork, stay left (right goes to Shannon Creek). At the second fork, about 100 metres farther, go left again (right goes to the Stawamus Squaw).

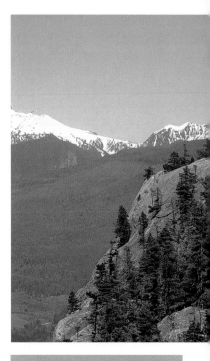

The Chief is essentially one rock, literally a monolith, which is believed to be about 93 million years old.

Fifteen minutes farther is a clearing with a view of a clearcut that is starting to grow back again. Continue along to the next fork in the trail and go left. Follow the orange diamonds and occasional red paint, which mark the way up. This part of the trail can be wet, so take care when clambering over rock or exposed tree roots. Use your hands for support and balance over the trickier spots.

Eventually, the trail leads under a massive chunk of granite overhanging the trail. Not much farther, the trail emerges from the forest to views and the beginning of a final scramble up bare rock.

At this point, you must make a decision, taking two things into consideration—the upcoming terrain and the current conditions. What lies ahead is bare rock covered in good part by moss and lichen, which means that even on the driest days the surface can be slippery. On wet days, sliminess is guaranteed.

Ask yourself and other members of your hiking party if you're comfortable with moving up exposed rock with potentially slippery conditions, or if you're content with the current views.

If you decide to continue, use caution. Don't hurry. Use your hands and feet as you follow the red paint marks to the peak. And if you come to a point where you're not comfortable, don't go further.

Once at the top, have a seat and take in the views of the Squamish Valley and peaks of the Tantalus Range and Garibaldi Park to the north, of the Centre and North summits to the northeast and of Howe Sound to the southwest.

And take comfort in the fact that the rock on which you're sitting isn't going anywhere fast. Kevin McLane spins the tale best in *Squamish, The Shining Valley*. According to McLane, the Chief was formed when dinosaurs still roamed the Earth, originating 30 kilometres below the surface as a huge blob of molten magma—the result of colliding continental plates. The magma was hotter and denser than the surrounding rock, rising and cooling gradually to a point about 10 kilometres below the surface. During that million-year period, the stresses and strains of cooling caused fractures. And into those conduits flowed hotter magma. It cooled rapidly and formed the sinuous black basalt dykes so beloved by rock-climbers.

Then, for millions of years, the forces of ice, water and earthquake eroded the earth above the Chief. When the Fraser glaciation began 25,000 years ago, the Chief had likely almost reached the earth's surface. As the glaciers ground south, they scoured the remaining softer rock from the Chief, creating the now-familiar shape. The gullies were gouged deeper and the great slabs of rock sheared off, leaving a tumble of massive boulders at the base. By about 10,000 years ago, most of the glaciers had retreated from the lowlands, and the Chief woke to the first light of day.

Once you've taken in the views, eaten lunch and are ready to head down, retrace your steps—feeling free to use your bum as a helper over the exposed rock—down to the forest floor, back to the bridge at Olesen Creek and to the parking lot at Shannon Falls.

STAWAMUS CHIEF: CENTRE & NORTH SUMMITS

36

Distance: 11 km	Rating: Moderate
Elevation gain: 500 m	Season: March to November
High point: 650 m	Topographical map:
Time needed: 5 hours	Squamish 92G/11
	Trail map: Page 167

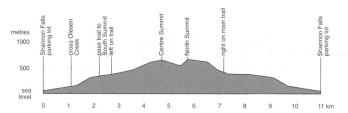

I F YOU'VE EVER BEEN TO SQUAMISH OR Whistler, you've passed the Chief. It's the enormous hunk of granite that looms a few hundred metres straight up.

In better weather, you can spot little blobs of colour on its surfaces; on closer inspection, you'll notice they're rock climbers. But you don't have to take the straight and vertical route to get to the top. There's a series of trails just behind the Chief that will take you to one, two or three of its peaks.

This hike covers two peaks—the Centre and the North summits—which see much less traffic than the popular South Summit. (Leave that peak for a cool, even overcast day, when fairweather hikers stay away in droves.)

Spring is the best time to hike the second and third peaks of the Chief. Any snow up top will likely be gone. And it's a good workout to get legs in shape for the stiffer hikes of summer.

To get to the trailhead, follow Highway 99 north towards Squamish. One kilometre past Shannon Falls Provincial Park, turn right at the first Stawamus Chief Provincial Park entrance. Stay right on the road to the walk-in campground. Park in the areas designated for non-campers.

Head for the park sign on the left of the road, and follow the trail through the campground to the sound of Olesen Creek and the start of the Stawamus Chief Trail.

Scramble up a rock outcrop and start your steady diet of uphill. From here, it's straight up on stone steps and wooden stairs. In a few minutes, a side-trail branches right to Shannon Falls park. Catch the views and your breath before tackling the next 30 to 40 minutes of uphill grunt.

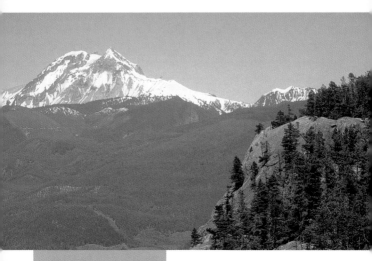

From the Centre Summit, you're in the middle of everything. The Squamish Valley and peaks of the Tantalus Range and of Garibaldi Provincial Park lie to the north. To the southwest is a grand view of the Chief's South Summit and of Howe Sound.

Go past the old logging paraphernalia, through the trees until you come to the bridge at Olesen Creek. Catch the views and your breath before tackling the next 30 to 40 minutes of steep uphill grunt.

At the first fork along the trail, stay left. (Right goes to Shannon Creek.) At the second fork, about 100 metres farther, go left again. (Right is the trail on which you'll return as well as the access to the Stawamus Squaw.) Continue to the next fork in the trail and go right. (Left goes to the South Summit.)

The trail for the 20 minutes or so can be a bit confused at times, so keep eyeballing the orange markers to stay on track. Eventually, the trail heads up a gully, then clambers up a rocky ledge, out of the forest and into the open. The bare rock here can be slippery, especially where moss or lichen has grown. Tread carefully and use your hands for balance.

Climb a sturdy but rickety-looking ladder and follow the orange slashes on the rock face to the summit. It's also a great vantage point to see the effects of glaciation on archetypal coastal terrain. Between 15,000 and 25,000 years ago, a vast sheet of ice poured down from the north scraping across mountain tops and gouging out great valleys. Here on the southwest coast of BC, it carved out Howe Sound, Indian Arm and Pitt Lake. At its height, the glacier measured 2000 metres thick and stretched as far south as Seattle.

When the climate began to warm, the ice melted and retreated north. In its wake, some of the valleys were first carved deeper by rivers of meltwater, and then filled. Some of the most southerly fjords in the Northern Hemisphere resulted, including Howe Sound.

After you've taken in the sights, had some lunch and a break, you can continue directly to the North Summit without backtracking, something you cannot do when going from the South Summit to the Centre Summit.

Keeping an eye on the orange markers, head north over the rock crest and descend into the saddle through the trees. Soon, you'll reach the North Gully with its unusual view of Mount Garibaldi. Stay north towards the top of the gully and prepare to scramble over rock again.

Head up onto a ledge and follow it to the end, then turn left and walk up a crest. The trail follows the orange markers to the right. Then, *voilà*, the North Summit with its little pond. From here, the views are northeast to the Stawamus Squaw and directly north to some of the Garibaldi Park peaks.

The rock on which you're sitting, by the way, is the same rock as that of the Centre and South summits. The Stawamus Chief is a monolith, literally one rock, just like the famous Ayers Rock in Australia's outback.

It's believed that the rock which makes up the Chief was first formed about 93 million years ago under the Earth's surface. Various geological processes such as uplift, intrusions, glaciation and erosion took place before the Chief raised the profile it shows today.

When you're ready to head homeward, backtrack to the North Gully and look for the trail heading farther downslope. The trail descends directly down the gully, winding around boulders and fallen logs, down, down, down to the forest floor.

At the bottom of the gully, head right and follow the trail to the bridge at Olesen Creek. Then retrace your steps to the parking area.

37 STAWAMUS SQUAW

Distance: 15 km

Elevation gain: 540 m

High point: 630 m

Time needed: 6 hours

Rating: Moderate

Season: March to November

Topographical map:
    Squamish 92G/11

Trail map: Page 167

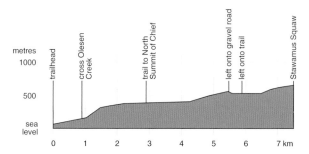

I F YOU'VE DRIVEN THE SEA TO SKY HIGHWAY, you know the Stawamus Chief. Its brooding profile rises 650 metres above the roadway in a sheer monolithic mass of granite—about 1.5 times the height of the world's tallest building.

The Chief's impressive bulk overshadows the town of Squamish and other lesser-known members of the 'family'— the Papoose, a smaller but distinct dollop of granite about a kilometre south of the Chief, and the Stawamus Squaw.

Every summer, more than 50,000 hikers tread their way along the trails behind the Chief to reach its first, second and third peaks. Far fewer folks venture farther into the Olesen Creek Valley to hike the Squaw. And that's a shame, not only because taking the less-travelled trail means more of the contemplative quiet that many hikers seek, but also because of the exquisite variety of scenery along the way.

To get to the trailhead, follow Highway 99 north towards Squamish. One kilometre past Shannon Falls Provincial Park, turn right at the first Stawamus Chief Provincial Park entrance. Stay right on the road to the walk-in campground. Park in the areas designated for non-campers.

Head for the park sign on the left of the road, and follow the trail through the campground to the sound of Olesen Creek and the start of the Stawamus Chief Trail.

Scramble up a rock outcrop and start the steady uphill. From here, it's straight up on stone steps and wooden stairs. In a few minutes, a side-trail branches right to Shannon Falls park. Catch

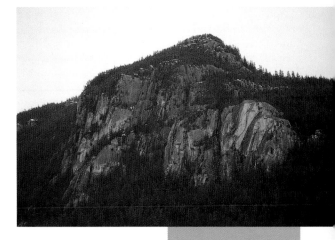

the views and your breath before tackling the next 30 to 40 minutes of uphill grunt.

Come here on a quiet weekday and you can avoid the heavy foot traffic that is inevitable most weekends—even wet ones!

At the first fork, stay left (right goes to Shannon Creek). At the second fork, about 100 metres later, go right (left goes to the Chief's south summit).

A forest fire lookout once stood on the summit, but now all that remains are bits of an old wood stove, some of the building timbers and fabulous views of Howe Sound, the Chief and the Squamish estuary to the west and Mount Habrich to the south.

The trail gets a bit confused at times because of recent blow-down, but just follow the orange markers and you'll come to another fork. This time, take the lower of the roads and go right. (The left and steeper route heads to the Chief's Centre and North summits.)

Within just a few minutes, you'll find yourself staring up at a long and massive cliff known to rock-climbers as 'The Cirque of the Uncrackables,' a play on the towers in the Yukon called 'The Cirque of the Unclimbables.' If you look closely, you'll see the silver-coloured bolts that mark routes with names like March of the Kitchen Utensils, Ivan Meets GI Joe and Magical Dog. What does it all mean? Only the original route climber knows for sure.

After the big walls come big trees—Douglas fir and western red cedar left uncut by early loggers—and then the first of the big views. A mossy rock bluff shows off sweeping views of the second-growth valley and a pretty waterfall cascading down the opposite ridge.

At a big rock, where the trail is a bit confusing, go down to the right. A bit farther along is another big wall with the 'bronto' tree—a big Douglas fir that has grown out and away from the base of the rock towards the light. From the near distance, it looks like a brontosaurus neck stretching from the bulk of its granite body.

About 100 metres farther is a sign: 'Trail closed due to erosion. Use new trail.' So, go right and follow the orange diamond markers to sun-kissed bluffs perfect for a water break and time to soak up the views.

Back on the trail, a few minutes of walking brings you to a swampy lake. Ten minutes beyond, look for a side-trail that leads to a bluff with a view of the Stawamus Chief not seen anywhere else. Follow the main trail as it gains elevation steadily and gradually through second-growth forest, then drops into a glade of alder, eventually emerging onto a rutted road.

Continue straight ahead, watching on the left for the pink tapes and small sign noting the side-trail to the Squaw. A quick scramble at the start and a bit of uphill soon brings you to a bluff looking southeast across the Stawamus River valley to Mount Mulligan.

From here, it's a mere 15 to 20 minutes to the summit. If you follow a short trail on the summit's backside to a viewpoint—with bench—you'll see the glacier-capped Mamquam Mountain shining in the east.

Glaciers once scoured the rock on which you're now perched. About 10,000 to 15,000 years ago, an ice sheet about 2000 metres deep covered southwestern BC. Until the climate began to warm and glaciers began to melt, only the highest peaks poked up above the icy surface.

When the glacier that carved out Howe Sound and the steep-walled slopes of the east side peaks retreated, huge gushing rivers poured forth. Smaller glaciers lingered in smaller valleys such as the Shannon Creek Valley. As Kevin McLane notes in *Squamish, The Shining Valley*:

> Around 10,000 years ago, the glacier in the Shannon Creek Valley would probably have retreated only as far as the top of the falls, where great towers of ice would peel off and crash 400 feet down the cascading waterfall.

When you're ready, just retrace your steps to the parking lot with a whole new perspective on Shannon Falls.

UPPER SHANNON FALLS `38`

Distance: 5 km return	Season: March to December
Elevation gain: 450 m	Topographical map:
High point: 500 m	Squamish 92 G/11
Time needed: 4 hours	Trail map: Page 167
Rating: Moderate	

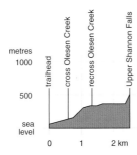

MOST PEOPLE ONLY SEE SHANNON FALLS from the bottom up. Most people only walk the couple hundred metres from the parking lot to the wooden stairways at the feet of BC's third-highest waterfall. But the sight up top where Shannon Creek begins its gravity-propelled descent is just as impressive.

The falls usually reach their peak in May, but the hike to upper Shannon Falls is good almost any time of the year, with the exception of the two coldest months. The trail is definitely a little trickier than the 200 metres of flat gravel trod by most people. With some sustained steep sections and lots of slippery surfaces, the hike to the upper falls is not for neophyte hikers. If you're new to day tripping, just be sure to go with a friend whose hiking boots have tramped many kilometres on tougher terrain.

To get to the trailhead, follow Highway 99 towards Squamish and watch for the BC Parks signs noting the turnoff to Shannon Falls Provincial Park. From the parking lot, head up the main pathway towards the falls. At the first fork, bear left to follow the sign pointing the way to the Stawamus Chief.

Where the trail forks, just past a 1925 steam donkey, go right. Other bits of old logging equipment line the trail as you follow the orange diamond markers put up by Federation of Mountain Clubs of BC crews. At the next fork, head right again. Soon, Olesen Creek comes into view, sometimes a trickle, other times swollen to a thundering tumble.

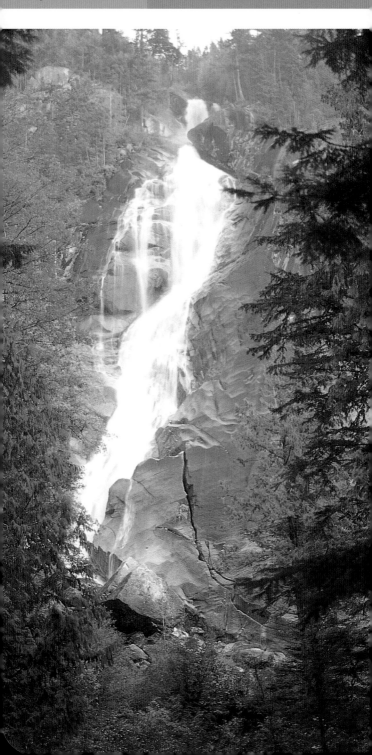

The bridge has good views of Howe Sound and the ever-changing hue of its waters. In spring, when snowmelt is pouring off nearby peaks, Howe Sound is a preternatural blue-green; in fall, when rain swells the Squamish River, the waters are rendered muddy and bobbing with debris.

The next section of trail is a 30- to 40-minute, steep uphill grunt, along sometimes slippery wood and rock, and through the occasional pocket of mud. Now that this section of trail falls within the new Stawamus Chief Provincial Park, some time and money is being spent to upgrade the trail. Finally, where the slog begins to level, just after a short section of boardwalk, the trail forks. Go right and into a grove of young hemlock trees (left goes to the Stawamus Chief trails).

A few minutes farther, the trail recrosses Olesen Creek. On the other side, the way can become slick and muddy at times. Just watch your step and take in the abundance of fern, fungi and other botanical life on the forest floor.

Soon, the stands of alder that line the path part for another view of Howe Sound and the snow-capped peaks across the way. Then it's time for the second uphill grunt, which winds quietly and steadily upward through a young forest of hemlock, cedar and the occasional western white pine. (Most western white pines were wiped out early in the 20th century after a fungus, called white pine blister rust, was accidentally imported into Vancouver from France in 1910.)

After 10 to 15 minutes of climbing upward, the trail levels. A spur trail to the right leads to a dawdling opportunity and another great view of Howe Sound. If you had happened to be hiking in, say 1792, you might have seen Captain George Vancouver's ship *Discovery* at anchor below in Darrell Bay. His journal describes the area:

> In this dreary and comfortless region, it was no inconsiderable piece of good fortune to find a little cove in which we could find shelter, and a small spot of level land on which we could erect our tent, as we had scarcely finished our examination when the wind became excessively boisterous from the southward attended by squalls and torrents of rain.

Well, Captain Vancouver may not have been a fan, but the famous winds from which Squamish takes its name (in the Coast Salish language, 'Sko-mish' means 'strong wind' or 'birthplace of the winds') are sought today by sailboarders who've made the Squamish Spit a mecca for windsurfing.

A few minutes of walking on level ground brings you to the beginning of another uphill grind, the steepest thus far. Wooden

Shannon Falls.

Sandwiched between the rock walls is a magical glade filled with cedars, fern-dripping boulders and a sense of uncommon tranquillity. It's easy to feel as if you had suddenly dropped into the pages of a fairy tale. The feeling lingers as you continue onward, tracing above the edges of a tiny rain-soaked pond. Decaying leaves of skunk cabbage visible under the water's surface are testimony to the pond's summertime existence as a marsh.

step ladders have been covered with chicken-wire to give boot treads a good grip, but other sections demand more attention. Take it slow or even stop for a moment to take in the beauty of some of the big trees in this section.

Fifteen minutes or so of huffing and puffing brings you to the best of the viewpoints so far. More open and less treacherous than the lower spot, this is a good place to stop for lunch before making the final push to the upper falls.

Once you're back on track, follow the trail as it noses down into a narrow canyon-like gully. Not much farther, the roar of the falls can be heard and the foaming white water glimpsed through a thin dark forest. Short spur paths dip off from the main trail for views of Shannon Creek as it rushes towards the precipitous plunge seen from ground level.

Keep a respectful distance and be extremely careful near the creek edge. A slip into this powerful maelstrom could be fatal.

The cascade below used to be known as Fairy Falls, which seems more in keeping with the feel of the trail. But, sometime around the beginning of the 20th century, it was renamed after William Shannon, a Squamish pioneer who lived nearby and manufactured bricks here before World War I. In the 1890s, Shannon also operated the largest hops farm in the Squamish Valley, near Brackendale. Squamish hops were reputed to be among the best in the world. Much of the crop was exported to Great Britain for beer-making.

Before retracing your steps to the trailhead, follow the marked trail upwards for five to 10 minutes to get a peek at Shannon Creek in its quieter moments, before it pitches and plunges through—and finally over—the stubborn granite that creates Shannon Falls.

SQUAMISH AREA

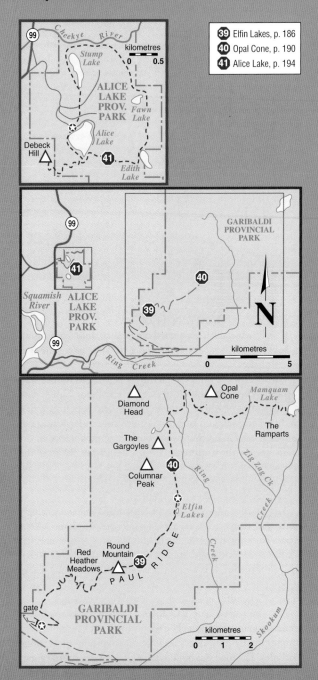

39 Elfin Lakes, p. 186
40 Opal Cone, p. 190
41 Alice Lake, p. 194

39 ELFIN LAKES

Distance: 22 km

Elevation gain: 600 m

High point: 1560 m

Time needed: 6 hours

Rating: Moderate

Season: July to October

Topographical map:
  Cheakamus River 92G/14 &
  Mamquam Mountain 92 G/15

Trail map: Page 185

Note: Dogs are not allowed in Garibaldi Provincial Park.

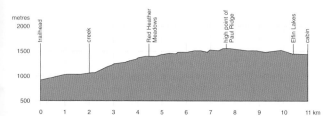

THE MOUNTAIN FOR WHICH GARIBALDI Provincial Park is named can be seen from many vistas, but the best views of the massif come along the trail to Elfin Lakes.

Garibaldi is not quite as splendidly isolated as it once was. Each year, the Diamond Head area attracts about 22,000 day-trippers, most of whom come in August and September, first for the wildflowers and later for the burnished tones of autumn. Your best bet for a less-crowded outing: go on a weekday.

To get to the trailhead, follow Highway 99 past the intersection to downtown Squamish, heading for Garibaldi Highlands and follow the BC Parks sign that marks the turnoff to Garibaldi Park–Diamond Head.

The paved road winds past the Squamish Golf and Country Club, and turns to gravel a bit farther on. At about 8 kilometres from the highway, the road forks. Stay left for another 5 kilometres to the parking lot. (Although the RCMP keeps an eye on the lot, it is a notorious venue for break-ins. Leave nothing inside; thieves have been known to smash a window to get at a handful of coins or a pair of sunglasses.)

Pass the yellow gate and follow an old access road as it gradually gains elevation. The way is lined with thimbleberry, stinging nettle and alder saplings that typically grow along roadsides. The road was built in the mid-1940s to shuttle guests to the old Diamond Head Lodge at Elfin Lakes. Now, however,

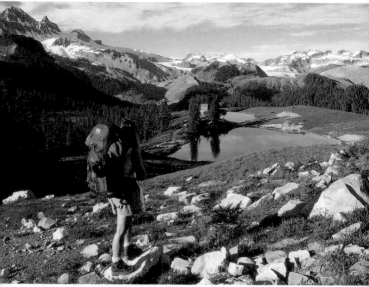

Atwell Peak, Elfin Lakes Trail.

it belongs to hikers, mountain bikers and the occasional BC Parks truck bringing in supplies.

Within 20 minutes, glimpses of the Tantalus Range can be seen through the trees. And soon after, there is a more open view, including that of the Squamish River below, all framed by lichen-draped mountain hemlock.

Now the plants along the trail are more blueberry bush, devil's club and first-growth forest. About 15 minutes farther, the road bends where a nameless creek tumbles down a rocky outcrop. It's a good place for a water break.

As you continue steadily uphill, the first hints of meadowy vegetation occur, such as blueberry bush, Labrador tea and, of course, red heather. Within 20 minutes of the creek, the first views of Mount Garibaldi appear. In autumn, with scarlet, ochre and gold alpine meadows in the foreground, it's a stunning sight.

Soon, you're in true subalpine with its ubiquitous meadows and ancient wizened trees. Pondlets are sprinkled everywhere. In summer months, the bugs here can be thick and fierce, pushing you faster towards the shelter that lets you know that you've arrived at Red Heather Meadows.

Just north of the shelter is a sign that tells a bit about the restoration work being done in the meadows. The subalpine environment with its thin soil and short growing season is a

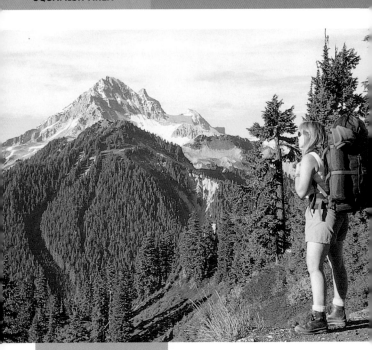

The ridge on which the lakes sit makes a perfect place to contemplate all the peaks and features that make up the Garibaldi massif: Atwell Peak on the south; an enormous wedge-shaped rock known as The Tent; and the true 2678-metre summit of Mount Garibaldi peeking out north.

fragile one. The result of all the visitors over the years has been erosion, soil compaction and deep gouges where hikers and bikers have gone off-trail. Restoration work started in 1989—trails were redirected, plants transplanted, rock dams and water bars built to slow down and redirect water. Slowly, the meadows are coming back. Just remember: look, don't trample.

Continue along to where big boulders block the road. Here, hikers go left for a scenic ramble through lush alpine meadow, and cyclists go right for a wider, rockier ascent. The hiking trail rises gently past aged yellow cedars, gnarled spruce and fir to a splendid view of Atwell Peak—the southern summit of Garibaldi. (The peak is also sometime incorrectly referred to as Diamond Head, but that name properly belongs to a the sloping shoulder just in front, Little Diamond Head.) Soon after, the trail rejoins the road. And the views open wide.

It's believed that, between 10,000 and 15,000 years ago, Mount Garibaldi was formed, as vast glaciers receded northward. The release of their weight on the land triggered intense volcanic activity; Garibaldi the volcano erupted with thick clouds of ash and burning rivers of lava. As the molten rock lapped over the retreating ice, billows of steam poured forth, rendering the perfect portrait of hell on Earth.

Mount Garibaldi today is cloaked year-round in a sheath of snow and ice. (The Squamish peoples called the mountain Cheekye, or 'Dirty Snow'.)

As the road levels, the cabins at Elfin Lakes become visible. And to the southeast, Mamquam Mountain rises into view. As the trail drops into a saddle, notice also the massive clearcut logging dead ahead. Some cuts go clear to the alpine—the same alpine environment that takes years to grow back just from being trodden on.

About 10 minutes farther is some consolation—a big, beautiful and ancient mountain hemlock on the left side of the trail. None of the timber on Paul Ridge has been cut, thanks to the efforts of early mountaineers and naturalists in getting the park set aside in 1927.

From here, the trail undulates along the ridge like long, slow swells. As it drops into the trough of one 'wave,' a vista slips from view; as it rises on the crest of the next wave, another view appears.

As the road begins its final descent, the two Elfin Lakes—once called Crystal Lakes—lie before you. Swimming is allowed in the upper lake; the lower is for drinking water only. In the near distance are the ranger's cabin, the overnight shelter and the old Diamond Head Lodge, closed since 1972 and now used for storage.

At the lower lakeside, a sign tells of the history of the lodge and the three people who made their dream of a little alpine idyll come true: West Vancouverite Joan Mathews and two Norwegian brothers, Emil and Ottar Brandvold.

If you're overnighting, there's a 34-bunk shelter and a campground 1 kilometre lower. Otherwise, just retrace your steps after a long, leisurely lunch.

40 OPAL CONE

Distance: 13 km
   (from Elfin Lakes)
Elevation gain: 250 m
High point: 1650 m
Time needed: 5 hours

Rating: Moderate
Season: July to September
Topographical map:
   Mamquam Mountain 92G/15
Trail map: Page 185

Note: Dogs are not allowed in Garibaldi Provincial Park.

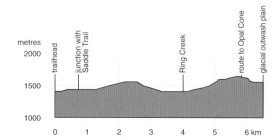

ANCIENT VOLCANOES, ETHEREAL GLACIER-fed lakes and moonscapes of rock, ice and snow are all an easy dayhike from Elfin Lakes. That means carrying a backpack with food and extra gear in from the Diamond Head parking area, or an overnight stay at either the Elfin shelter or the campground in the meadows 1 kilometre below. But it's a small effort to make in order to see some truly wow terrain.

Starting from the Elfin Lake shelter, follow the trail north to the junction with the Campground Trail. Keep on going through an alpine meadow that in summer is filled with wildflowers. In September, the blooms are gone, but the foliage of blueberry bushes and other shrubs burns brightly in the autumn light.

Within 10 minutes, the trail reaches a junction where the signpost looks as though it has been used as a scratching or chewing post by some of the neighbourhood bruins. Continue straight ahead on level trail in the direction of Mamquam Lake. (The Saddle Trail goes left to a saddle visible in the near distance.)

Soon, the trail descends to a feeder creek. Recent slide action may cover part of the trail with mud, rock and a displaced mountain hemlock or two. A few minutes farther is another creek. In early summer, the meltwater can really howl through here. But by fall, it has dwindled to a trickle.

The trail heads gently upward for a stretch, then levels, then drops again, this time towards Ring Creek, the waterway that

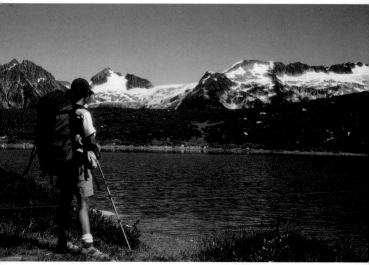

The Mamquam Massif.

all the other creeks feed into. An ancient glacier carved out the trough before you. Moraine ridges can be seen higher up the western slopes of Opal Cone where debris was deposited by an ice sheet as it ground forward.

In the distance, you can see the trail ahead worn into the outwash plain. Ring Creek rushes below, fed even in fall by constant meltwater from the permanent icefields on high.

Even the geology along the trail here is interesting. Note especially the ancient lava flows cooled instantly into basalt columns as they hit the glacier. It looks as if someone has intentionally stacked perfectly fitted blocks into platforms for some unknown purpose.

In summer, wildflowers—Indian paintbrush, lupine, fireweed—line the trail as you descend to the 'Please follow arrows' rock. From here, the way is rocky and open and can be blazing hot in full sun. Follow the cairns and pieces of orange-daubed broomstick, which mark the first crossing of Ring Creek. The rocks are usually slimy, so watch your footing as you boulder-hop across. It's also a good spot for a water break.

The trail continues up across the old moraine, beautiful in a barren way. To the west are clear views of Little Diamond Head and Atwell Peak and the aptly named Gargoyles, likely ancient volcanic vents plugged with rock harder than that which eroded away. Directly ahead is Opal Cone.

Follow the bits of broomstick handle down to the next arm of the creek and cross over the bridge. On the other side,

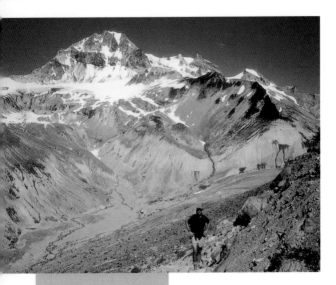

Occasionally, the trail passes trees that are huge for this elevation. In the subalpine, the soils are thin and the growing season short, so trees don't have the time to grow as big and tall as the ones lower in the valley. Here, the mountain hemlocks may look kind of average, but if you were to count the rings within, you'd see layers of cambium so thin that they look like onionskin.

pick up the trail by the now-familiar orange-broomstick markers and head up, steeply at first, then gradually but steady. About 10 minutes farther, the trail switchbacks sharply to the southeast and traverses the moraine ridge.

Ten minutes farther is the high point of the ridge with views southeast to the Mam-quam Mountain and south to extensive logging cuts. Follow the Opal Cone sign into a beautiful, lush green bowl, being sure to make noise for any bears in the vicinity. In summer, the meadows here are thick with wildflowers. In fall, towhead babies (western anemones gone to seed) bob their moptops with the slightest breeze. The trail leads through the cool respite of an alpine grove and up a small slope, eventually reaching a trail junction.

Here, you must decide whether to explore the upper reaches of Opal Cone, which involves some scrambling and route-finding, or whether to explore the icy green lake and the glacial moraine straight ahead.

If you opt for Opal Cone, go left and uphill to follow the path as it balances on the top of an old moraine ridge. At the end of the ridge, you can see a similar lakelet visible just behind the first, as well as the toe of the Lava Glacier.

Past this point, the trail is not marked. And you must now scramble up a steep slope of loose dirt. Soon the pitch lets up. Follow the occasional cairn up the gully on the right. Just past a big crumbly boulder, the trail bears left. At a monster boulder, its surface striated by a glacier, it's a short scramble to the cairn up top that marks the high point.

You are literally sitting on the rim of an ancient volcano that blew its insides out. And the views are 360° of wow. To the southwest is the Elfin Shelter, Columnar Peak and the Gargoyles. To the west is Diamond Head, Atwell Peak and Mount Garibaldi. The Diamond Glacier spills off Atwell. To the north is the Garibaldi Névé; the tongue of Garibaldi Glacier slides west of Opal Cone and Lava Glacier slides east. To the southeast is Pyramid Mountain and the Mamquam Massif.

If you decide to continue straight on from the junction, there are hours of exploring that can be done on the moraine—a veritable moonscape of lava, granite and greenstone pummeled by the ice into a broad sheet of rock debris. Occasional boulders dot the landscape where the glacier left them behind.

Some moss, grass and hardier plants provide green patches. Eventually, vegetation may overtake the area and alpine meadows may regrow—unless the next ice age happens first.

The trail eventually cuts between two ponds used by resident wildlife, as evidenced by the black bear, coyote and other tracks in the mud. From here, the trail drops down to the banks of Zig Zag Creek, then climbs up to the Ramparts— a two-hour return trip. From the top of the Ramparts, you can see Mamquam Lake tucked below but it's a long way down and an even longer way up.

For the return—whether you decide to scramble up Opal Cone, explore the glacial plain or extend the trip to the Ramparts—just retrace your steps back to Elfin Lakes. And be sure to let the bears know you're coming home.

41 ALICE LAKE PROVINCIAL PARK

Distance: Up to 12 km	Season: Year-round
Elevation gain: Minimal	Topographical map:
High point: 400 m	Cheakamus River 92G/14
Time needed: Up to 4 hours	Trail map: Page 185
Rating: Easy	Note: Dogs must be leashed.

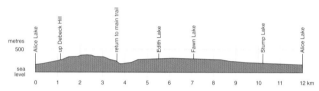

S PRING IS POSSIBLY THE BEST TIME TO explore the lakes and trails of Alice Lake Provincial Park, but Alice Lake is also a good destination for the short days of winter and the less-crowded days of fall. The only time to avoid this popular 400-hectare park just north of Squamish is summer, when crowds descend on the campground and tiny beaches.

There are two options to this outing. The shorter two-hour circuit connecting the park's four lakes is good for less-than-perfect weather or for families looking for a kid-friendly destination. The longer four-hour trip, which includes Debeck Hill, can make for a good winter workout or easy spring training for the longer, steeper hikes of summer to come.

The starting point for both hikes is the main parking lot at the park. To get there, head north on Highway 99 past Squamish, past Brackendale and take the turnoff leading east to Alice Lake Provincial Park. As you enter the park proper, continue past the campground turnoff and park near the big map and bathrooms at Alice Lake.

Wander down to the shores of the lake and follow the tree-fringed trail to the right along the western shore. In just a few minutes, you'll emerge onto another beach. To follow the old road to the top of Debeck Hill, continue straight south towards a yellow gate. Then follow the small brown sign noting the steady uphill way.

About 30 minutes along is a remnant of the railway logging done here in the 1940s—an old steam donkey (a piece of

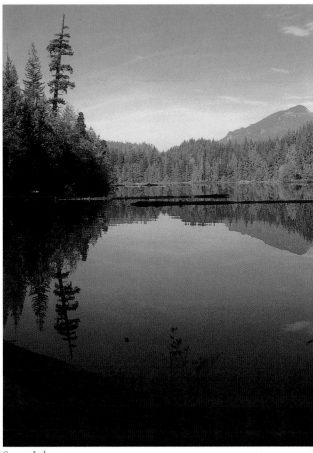

Stump Lake.

early logging equipment, used for hauling logs down slopes), remarkably intact despite the rust and wood rot.

Another 20 minutes of uphill hiking on loose rock road brings you to the top of the hill, where the scenery is marred by no fewer than three antennae towers. Still, on a clear day, the views of the Squamish River and the Tantalus Range are worth every step.

Descending the trail will bring you back to the south shore beach of Alice Lake, named after Squamish pioneer Alice Rose, who settled in the area with her husband Charles in the late 1800s. Cross the parking lot to the big Four Lakes Trail sign and head right, to follow the path as it winds alongside Edith Creek. Mountain bikers share these trails, and although they're supposed to yield right of way to hikers, it's best to stay alert.

About 15 to 20 minutes later is Edith Lake, the first of the three tiny lakes tucked away from the bustle surrounding Alice. In 1890, the Merrill and Ring Lumber Company from Seattle acquired a chunk of timber from the provincial government stretching from Alice Lake south to the Stawamus Chief. The price was 25 cents per acre. In 1926, Merrill and Ring began logging the area, and after 14 years of cutting and hauling only the biggest and best trees, the company made, undoubtedly, a hefty profit on its investment.

> The trail rises gently through denser moss-covered forest to the top of a small ridge on which you'll amble under the more open boughs of second-growth western hemlock, western red cedar and the occasional western white pine.

Keep left to continue to Fawn Lake (right leads outside the park boundaries). At an intersection about five minutes farther, cross the well-travelled dirt road to pick up the trail opposite. If you encounter a yellow caution sign, you're going the wrong way. Turn right to connect with the trail proper.

Ten minutes later is a yellow gate. Circumnavigate any seasonal mud puddles and go left through the gate and onto a short side-trail to the shores of Fawn Lake, a pretty little waterhole with a tiny beach that is perfect for a rest break.

After contemplating Fawn's peace and quiet, head back to the main trail and bear left to continue to Stump Lake. Within a few minutes, the path trundles through a chunk of forest thinned by significant blowdown. From here, the first rushings of the Cheekye River can be heard. Eventually, the trail winds down to river level. During the spring freshets, the tiny Cheekye can really howl.

Heading away from the river, the trail comes to the north end of Stump Lake. Go right to take the slightly higher part of Stump's loop trail with its scenic views of lake, mountain and forest. As the trail nears the end of the lake, continue straight until you reach the paved road. Cross and go past the yellow gate and straight down the hill through the campground. When you can see the shores of Alice Lake, you need only bear right to bring you to the starting point at the big park sign.

SEA TO SKY CORRIDOR

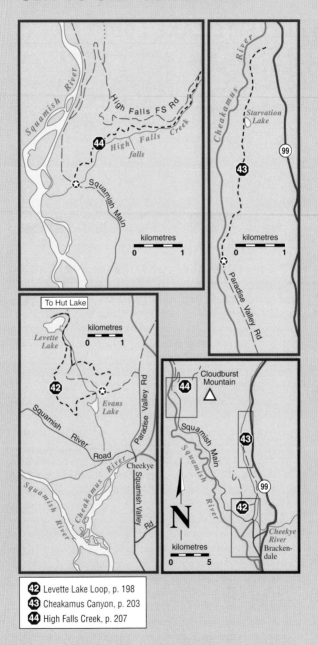

42 Levette Lake Loop, p. 198
43 Cheakamus Canyon, p. 203
44 High Falls Creek, p. 207

42 LEVETTE LAKE LOOP

Distance: 11 km	Rating: Easy to moderate
Elevation gain: 300 m	Season: April to November
High point: 400 m	Topographical map:
Time needed: 5 hours	Cheakamus River 92G/14
	Trail map: Page 197

Note: Do not trespass on the Evans Lake Forestry Camp.

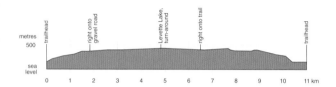

S OMETIMES, YOU'VE HAD A LONG WEEK, AND then the weekend comes. You want to get out into the great outdoors for a scenic hike, but you just don't have the kind of energy it takes to do a long, steep epic. Sometimes, you want the views, the variety and the feeling of getting away from it all—in just a few hours of easy hiking. Such a place can be found in the Levette Lake area, just north of Squamish.

Here, for relatively little effort expended, are splendid views of the Tantalus Range to the west, Garibaldi to the east, and the Squamish River valley to the south. As well, there's Levette Lake where you can eat your lunch and soak your toes.

To get to the trailhead, drive north on Highway 99 past Squamish, past Brackendale to the turnoff leading to Cheekye. Turn left and follow the Squamish Valley Road through Cheekye and over the bridge. Immediately, the road forks. Go right and follow Paradise Valley Road to the big sign noting the North Vancouver Outdoor School. Turn left onto the road directly opposite. Parts are paved, parts are gravel, but most vehicles will have no problem covering the kilometre or so to the next fork, marked by an Evans Lake Forestry Camp sign. Park off the road in the pullouts. Slip on your boots and follow a path on the right (east side) leading uphill into the trees.

A signboard shows all the trails in the area and gives information about the forest through which you'll hike. The trail that follows an old skid road up to Copperbush Pond, for example, goes through a stand of juvenile trees, planted in 1955 and spaced for less-crowded, optimal growing conditions in 1963. Make some mental notes, then head off up the steepish skid road.

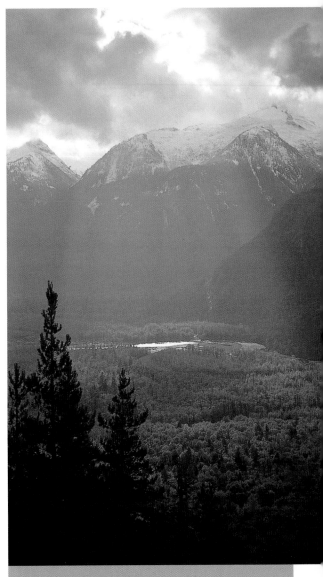

The Squamish River snaking through the wide wash of the
valley is only the end run of water that began as trickles from
melting glaciers and snowpack high in the mountains of the
Pemberton Icecap. The river traces the route of a vast glacier
that scoured the valley long ago.

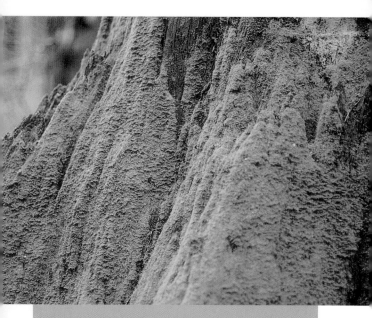

A verdant layer of preternaturally green moss gives new life to an old stump. About 700 species of true mosses blanket the southern coast, from the tiny branchlets of tree moss to the spindly stems of tall-clustered tree moss. While mosses cover a spectrum of green from pale jade to deep emerald, there are also species coloured as black as charred toast (black rock moss, also known as granite moss) and red like flames (red roof moss, also known as fire moss).

Like other nonvascular plants—those with tissues that don't conduct water and food as well as tissues of vascular plants such as trees, flowers and ferns—mosses thrive in wet places. Some species of moss that live in dry places have the ability to survive a drying out. When they become wet again—usually through rainfall—their photosynthesis mechanism kicks into gear once again.

Some moss species were used by Native Peoples in making dyes and medicines. And in the forest ecosystem, mosses play an important role in allowing trees such as maple, alder and cottonwood to extract water and nutrients from moss pads and nitrogen-fixing lichens.

Ten to 15 minutes later, the road levels and a side-trail branches east to Silver Summit, a route that's best left for another day. Continue left through the young forest punctuated with big stumps to reach the side-trail leading to Copperbush Pond.

On its swampy shores sits a quaint wooden shelter. The pond, only a block long and hemmed in by vegetation, may not be the highlight of the hike, but it's pretty in its own close, quiet way. Back on the main trail, continue north through marshy sections and a section of forest that can be quite dense and dark unless sunlight filters through.

Soon, the trail emerges to more open terrain and leads up a gully, under a big rock wall and across a slimy, rotting wooden bridge before traversing west then up to a rocky bluff.

After the mini-grunt, it's worth stopping for a water break and to check out the views of the Cheakamus River and the peaks of Garibaldi Park to the east. Once you've rested, follow the trail west and down into a gully. Notice how the forest has changed? This section of the trail passes through untouched old-growth. Among the moss-covered boulders and rocky outcrops grow big trees, including a very special little grove of Douglas fir—one of the most beautiful parts of the hike.

The trail climbs through a cleft in the rock and wanders across ancient mossy rockfalls before scrambling up a rock outcrop and continuing gently upwards farther into the forest. For 20 to 30 minutes, the trail continues, sometimes over rockfalls now overgrown with salal, alder and cedar saplings until it finally arrives at a wooden bridge and then the old logging road to Levette.

If you've had enough, descend the logging road back to your vehicle. Otherwise, continue up the road, eventually crossing a wooden bridge (which also marks the trail you'll pick up on the return) and, farther, a sign indicating 'No Power Boats' near a green outhouse. On the left are bluffs on which you can clamber down to the shore of Levette Lake, find a picnic spot and relax.

When you're ready to continue, retrace your steps along the logging road to just before the wooden bridge. A trail slides off to the right; follow the old logging road through a dense growth of alder for about 15 to 20 minutes. The Skyline Trail takes off to the left. Although it's marked by red arrows, the trail can be overgrown at times, so keep a close eye on the markers as the path winds its way onto a ridge. Your reward: stunning views of the Tantalus Range and the Squamish River valley.

The Tantalus Range was named by early mountaineer Neal Carter to whom the peaks suggested the legend of

King Tantalus. In Greek mythology, Tantalus was a king and lower-level deity who was intimate friends with the god Zeus. Zeus often invited the demi-deity to Olympian banquets, but Tantalus got a little greedy and stole nectar and ambrosia to share among his mortal buddies. For that and a couple of other godly transgressions, Tantalus was condemned to dangle for eternity from the bough of a fruit-tree, which leaned over a marshy lake, and to suffer perennial thirst and hunger. (Whenever he would bend to drink from the lake, the waters would recede from his cupped hands. When he reached out to pluck the pears, apples, figs, pomegranates and dates that rubbed against his shoulders, a wind would blow them from his grasp.)

After absorbing the views, continue across the ridge and follow the trail. At one point, a flight of steps cuts into a fallen log in its steep descent to a gully. Now you'll go up again, through an overgrown bit of trail (again) to another viewpoint, this time with views of the peaks of Garibaldi Park to the east.

The trail traverses the ridge through thick masses of knee-high salal and head-high conifers to another viewpoint with more great views of the Tantalus Range. Stop and listen to the silence, interrupted only by the rumble of the Squamish River below and the trickle of a waterfall in the distance.

Then descend in the direction of the red triangles and a few minutes later emerge to the Fraser Burrard Trail. Go right and follow the path through the trees for 30 minutes or so to a granite monolith with a view that's worth looking at, if not quite as wow as the earlier vistas. Then descend to flat land and cross a small creek to the end of the Fraser Burrard.

The Evans Lake Forestry Camp is visible on the right, but do not trespass on this private property. Instead, ascend a slight hill on the left perimeter to emerge once again on the logging road. From here, it's only 200 metres downhill to your car.

CHEAKAMUS CANYON 43

Distance: 9 km	Season: February to November
Elevation gain: 200 m	Topographical map:
High point: 400 m	Cheakamus River 92G/14
Time needed: 3 hours	Trail map: Page 197
Rating: Easy	

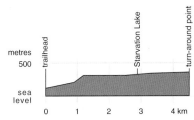

G LACIER-SWEPT PEAKS, DRAMATIC ROCK bluffs and canyon views are part of what's made Highway 99 such a popular drive between Squamish and Whistler. But some of the best sights can't be seen from the road. For them, you need a good pair of hiking boots.

The Cheakamus Canyon has long been used as a route for travel, first by the Squamish and Lillooet peoples to trade goods, later by gold-seekers and even, briefly, by ranchers driving cattle south. Now it is part of the Sea to Sky Trail, an ambitious project to provide a 150-kilometre off-road route from D'Arcy to Squamish for hikers, mountain bikers and horseback riders.

To get to the trailhead, follow Highway 99 past Squamish and Brackendale. At the last intersection before the road speeds to Whistler, turn left towards Cheekye. Follow the Squamish Valley Road across the bridge over Cheekye River and immediately afterward, turn right onto Paradise Valley Road. Zero your odometer, then follow the road over the single-lane bridge across the Cheakamus River. At 5.7 kilometres, the road turns to gravel. Follow it along under the powerlines to cross another wooden single-lane bridge. At 9.7 kilometres is a Y-junction; stay right. The next 1.7 kilometres can be rough. Go as far as you can and park in one of the pullouts just before the road ends in a washout.

The next 1.5 kilometres of road is rough and requires a four-wheel drive vehicle. You could also bring a bicycle. Otherwise, add another 3 kilometres and 45 minutes to the hike. The road trundles through mud and thickets of alder and brush to emerge alongside the Cheakamus River.

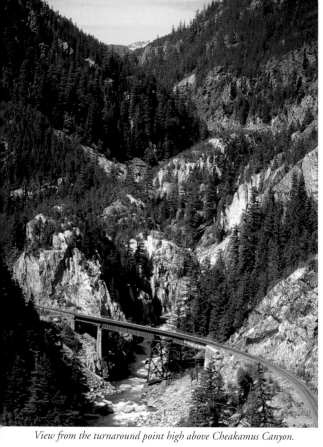

View from the turnaround point high above Cheakamus Canyon.

Eleven kilometres from Cheekye, the road disintegrates into a washout.

Take a moment to dawdle at the edge of the river. Its name, by the way, is a Coast Salish word meaning roughly 'place where they fish for salmon with cedar weirs.'

Follow the pink ribbons uphill into a copse of alder, then through a section of rockfall. While you're hiking up, notice the rocks underfoot. Most are familiar salt-and-pepper granite, but there are also red and black rocks—old lava, some pocked with air bubbles.

The road then levels out to a wide road under a canopy of second-growth red alder, western hemlock and the occasional western red cedar. Peaks of the Tantalus Range are visible to the west. All too soon, there's another uphill section, which will bring you to the railway tracks. Cross carefully to the dirt mound on the other side, marked by orange tapes.

The path enters the forest again alongside a pretty gully lush with growth. It then heads uphill once again, over more rockfall, and onto the remnant of an old lava flow, likely from Mount Garibaldi when it blasted into being between 10,000 and 15,000 years ago.

The trail soon levels out into a wide road again and shortly hugs the western shore of Starvation Lake, so named, we can only guess, by a disappointed fisherman. As you take a lakeside break, look over to the rocky ridge above the eastern shore. Just on the other side is Highway 99. All this comprises terrain that was formidable to early settlers who sought to establish a road between Squamish and the farming and ranching community of Pemberton.

In 1858, Governor James Douglas sent two men from Lillooet to scout out a route to Howe Sound that would be less harrowing and less troublesome than the established routes gold-seekers already took through the Fraser Canyon, along Harrison and Anderson Lakes. The pair made it out, but the governor ruled out the route as too difficult.

The area saw little travel until 1873, when William Samson was engaged to begin surveying and constructing a cattle trail. The cost, first estimated at $8000, ballooned to $37,000 by 1877, amid charges, according to Kevin McLane in *Squamish, the Shining Valley,* of 'contractors lining their pockets, bobbery and incompetence.'

The path continues downhill and crosses a makeshift bridge of log and rock, then heads uphill. The full roar of the Cheakamus River filters in and as the road winds along the east side bluffs, the peaks of the canyon can be seen. Tiny lodgepole pine and Douglas fir trees cling to the rock face and line the way like a quarry garden. Rotting ancient timbers keep rockfall from spilling onto the railway tracks below.

Just beyond is the first great view of the Cheakamus River and Canyon in steep, stunning glory. Twin waterfalls cascade around a large mid-river boulder, and below, a massive railway bridge hugs the precipitous slope.

This area was described by William Samson in 1873 as 'very rough, passing over rock slides or bluffs of solid rock.' Despite the difficulties, the trail—called Pemberton Cattle Trail, Squamish Trail, Howe Sound Trail or Burrard-Lillooet Trail—was completed in 1877.

That September, the first and only cattle drive on the trail took place. Rancher Robert Carson and two cowhands drove 200 head of cattle through bad weather along a route scarce in vegetation for feed but ample in troublesome terrain. During the last few kilometres, it is said, many of the weakened cattle fell off the steep trail or were lost in deep snow. (The men eventually did reach their destination. The cattle were sold and overwintered in the Fraser Valley to fatten them up.)

Fortunately, your going is easier as you continue up a gentle incline and across a big jumble of rockfall with good views across to the opposite bluff with its hoodoo-like pinnacle. Soon, the path leads to a big moss-covered rock outcrop, which in July and August is scattered with wildflowers. To the southwest are more views of the Tantalus Range.

The road leads gently upward through a narrow slot in the rock. Ten minutes farther is an ancient rockfall strewn with fallen trees and a big Douglas fir that has survived all the rockslides.

A few minutes later, the trail rounds a bluff with northward views of the upper canyon, the railway bridge that crosses the river and, in the distance, the traffic of Highway 99. Make this your turnaround point. If you're fortunate, a train may pass over the bridge as you munch your lunch.

After the failed cattle drive, the Howe Sound Trail went pretty much unused except by hardier individuals who travelled on horseback to transport goods, or as in the case of Whistler pioneers Alex and Myrtle Philip, for a 1910 fishing holiday. Two years later, a route for the Pacific Great Eastern Railway was surveyed. In 1918, the first train whistled through.

When you're ready to move on, simply retrace your steps—mostly downhill now—to your starting point on the Cheakamus River.

HIGH FALLS CREEK 44

Distance: 7–12 km	Season: May to October
Elevation gain: 650 m	Topographical map:
High point: 725 m	Cheakamus River 92G/14
Time needed: 4–5 hours	Trail map: Page 197
Rating: Moderate	

Note: This is a steep and exposed trail **not** recommended for children or adults with a fear of heights.

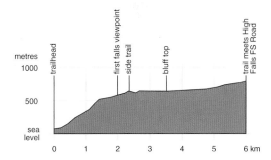

T HE TRAIL TO HIGH FALLS IS ONE OF THE most scenic hikes between Squamish and Whistler. From this trail are superb views of the Squamish River valley and the Tantalus Range, as well as of the High Falls themselves.

But this is not a hike for everyone. It runs at times not far from the cliff edge of an extremely steep canyon. A simple slip, which might, in other places, result in a bruised bum or a sore arm, could lead here to a long, deadly fall. (In fact, in 1994, a young woman who was part of an experienced hiking group did slip and fall to her death.)

It is definitely **not** a hike for kids. And, if you are at all uncomfortable with heights or clambering up steep exposed slopes, it is likely not for you either. That said, it is a lovely trail. Just one on which caution is required.

To get to the trailhead, follow Highway 99 north past Squamish and Brackendale. At the last intersection before the road continues to Whistler, turn left towards Cheekye. Follow the Squamish Valley Road across the bridge over Cheekye River, stay left and zero your odometer.

About 20 kilometres farther, the Squamish Valley Road turns to gravel for a 2-kilometre section, then pavement. At kilometre 22.6, you'll pass the powerhouse. At kilometre 23.4 is

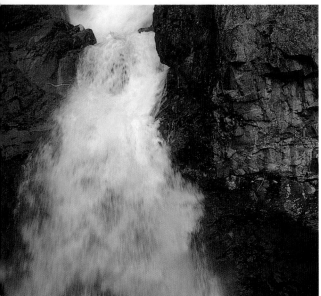

High Falls.

High Falls Creek. Park in the wide gravel pullouts on this side of the creek.

Cross the bridge on foot and head up the road for about 25 metres towards a fluttering strand of orange tape and a High Falls Creek Trail sign. Go right to follow an old logging road that in autumn can be barely visible under all the fallen broadleaf maple leaves.

With the sound of the creek on the right, the trail leads to the foot of a bluff. Scramble up to the blufftop with the first views of the day, only 10 to 15 minutes from the vehicle. On clear days, peaks of the Tantalus Range are visible across the valley, itself a sea of alder, cottonwood, maple and young conifers.

Continue scrambling up using the braided plastic rope for help. The trail climbs through a small grove of lodgepole pine, western hemlock and Douglas fir—some clinging precariously to the cliff edge.

Just beyond a big rock outcrop is another steep section with braided rope and, a few minutes farther, a side-trail that makes a short jaunt to another bluff top for even bigger views. In May, mountain goats can occasionally be seen on the slopes directly above the west side of the river (yes, the impossibly steep-looking slopes).

Back on the main trail, you'll soon come to a point that affords a precipitous view across to the steep walls of the canyon's south side, which was first surveyed by master trailbuilder Halvor Lunden for a trail to High Falls. Thankfully, he also scoped out the less-steep north side, and in 1957, built his first trail in BC.

The forest all along the trail is magnificently mature with an open understorey of salal and fern and big trees. Because it lies in such steep terrain, it's never been logged.

The trail veers away from the cliff edge for a bit then returns to climb along moss-covered bluffs. Across the way, a small waterfall trickles down the steep granite falls. And from farther upstream comes the first thundering sounds of the higher falls.

Soon, there's another steep, exposed section to clamber up—without a braided rope. At the top, a side-trail branches right to the first viewpoint of High Falls. From here, a white veil of water ricochets off a step and cascades to the unseen chasm below. You can hear the full roar of the water as it hits the bottom, but you can't see it, so don't even think of craning your head over the steep cliff edge.

Once back on the main trail, continue up. Soon, there's another steep section, with a braided rope to help get you to the top of another bluff. A side-trail leads left to vast views of the Squamish River valley and floodplain stretched below. The Tantalus Range forms a formidable, glacier-swept backdrop.

The main trail continues through a grove of tiny trees along the bluff top. Another short side-trail leads left to a big old Douglas fir and more valley views. To the right is an even more stunning view of the falls: the water plummeting from above, slamming against the wall opposite, then squeezing in a plume to a lower seat before leaping to the canyon below.

Bear left to clamber up two more bluff viewpoints and a third look at the falls, including a view of the car-sized boulder wedged mid-chute, past which the water must squeeze. Climb through a notch in the next bluff to quite possibly the most-ravishing viewpoint of all—a large green moss-carpeted bluff with wide open views of the river and mountains.

From here, the trail eases somewhat and rambles across mossy bluffs and into the trees. Where the trail enters the forest is a big Douglas fir about 40 metres high and punctuated with woodpecker holes.

The trail climbs upward to reach a junction where a side-trail branches right to a viewpoint beside the falls—just above where the car-sized boulder sits. Although you can't see the long plume below, you can hear thundering water and see the

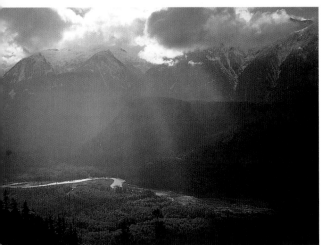

View of Squamish Valley and Tantalus Ridge from High Falls.

smooth round walls that the water has carved out over the ages. (Just stay away from the cliff edge; it's slippery, crumbly and if you slip, it's certain death.)

Once back at the main trail, traverse an old rockfall under a menacing bluff that seems ready to join the rock underfoot at any moment. A braided rope helps you over a bare rock face now used by an opportunist stream as its bed. The path climbs up to a steep-sided gully filled with big hemlock and fir, then sashays onto a southside bluff.

Climb steadily through a magical grove of old-growth forest and, 10 minutes farther, take the side-trail right to a bluff top with views that threaten to knock your boots right off. To the south/southwest is the Squamish River valley and the Tantalus Range peaks—Pelion, Ossa and Zenith mountains, as well as Mounts Tantalus and Dione. To the east is Cloudburst Mountain and, to the northeast, a nameless 1825-metre peak.

It's the perfect perch for lunch and a good turnaround point. If, however, you want to ramble farther or if you think you'd feel uncomfortable taking the steeper way down, continue along the trail through mature forest for another 15 minutes to reach a poorly marked junction. The left trail leads to the logging road about 10 to 15 minutes distant. The right trail continues farther through the forest to emerge higher up the logging road.

If you follow the logging road back down to the Squamish Mainline, you'll get great views to north Squamish Valley. But you'll also have a 1.5-kilometre walk back along the main logging road to your vehicle.

SEA TO SKY CORRIDOR

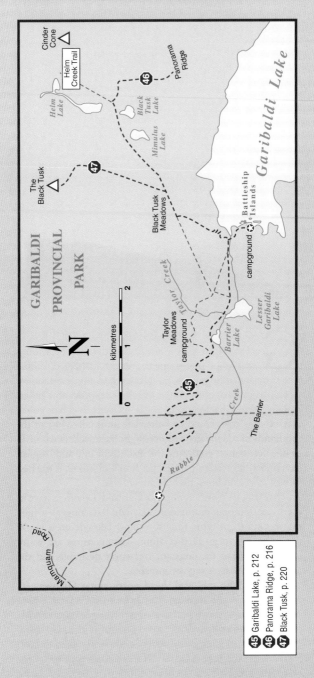

Cinder Cone

Helm Creek Trail

46

Panorama Ridge

Helm Lake

Black Tusk Lake

Mimulus Lake

Garibaldi Lake

The Black Tusk

47

Black Tusk Meadows

Battleship Islands

campground

GARIBALDI PROVINCIAL PARK

Taylor Creek

Lesser Garibaldi Lake

N

Taylor Meadows campground

Barrier Lake

kilometres

0 1 2

45

Barrier Creek

The Barrier

Rubble Creek

Mamquam Road

45 Garibaldi Lake, p. 212
46 Panorama Ridge, p. 216
47 Black Tusk, p. 220

45 GARIBALDI LAKE

Distance: 18 km	Rating: Moderate
Elevation gain: 810 m	Season: July to October
High point: 1450 m	Topographical map:
Time needed: 6 hours	Cheakamus River 92G/14
	Trail map: Page 211

Note: Be sure to wear sturdy hiking boots and carry lots of water.
You'll need both.

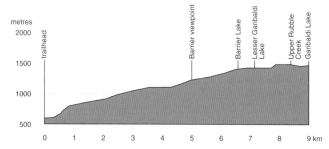

GARIBALDI LAKE, IN HIKING CIRCLES, IS what's known as a classic. At the end of a long-established trail is superb scenery—a large turquoise lake surrounded by mountains, glaciers and alpine meadows.

Garibaldi Lake is also often the choice of first-time hikers and overnight backpackers, so if solitude is what you're craving, this trail would be better left until fall. Most of the thousands of dayhikers and overnight backpackers who trip to this destination go during the months of July and August. September, says senior park ranger Ron Goldstone, is the best month to go: no bugs, no kids, no crowds.

That said, it's worth noting that Garibaldi Lake does have its merits as a summer destination. Daylight lasts longer—which means you've got more time to explore lakeside or, if you're overnighting, to go farther afoot. Temperatures are warm enough to make the constant tree-cover desirable and the lake's coolish waters very swimmable.

To get to the trailhead, head north along Highway 99 past Squamish, and through the Cheakamus Canyon. About 35 kilometres from Squamish, watch for the familiar BC Parks sign, which signals the upcoming turnoff to Garibaldi Park–Black Tusk. Just past Rubble Creek, turn right and drive 3 kilometres to the parking lot. (Note that this parking lot has one of the highest numbers of break-ins in the province. Leave nothing in your vehicle to tempt thieves.)

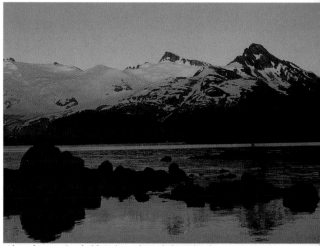

Alpenglow on Garibaldi Lake and Battleship Islands.

At the southeast corner of the upper lot the trail begins, leading directly into the cool of the forest alongside Rubble Creek. The ascent begins almost immediately. From here on, the way leads steadily and relentlessly upward.

A wide trail winds through a forest of mostly Douglas fir and hemlock supported by pockets of devil's club, which is at times both monstrous and impenetrable. Big, beautiful red cedars begin to appear about 25 minutes later. Then comes a small wooden bridge over a creek—the only source of water that you'll see for almost two long, hot hours. So dunk the hat, soak the bandanna and push on.

About 20 minutes farther up the trail is a white post noting the 3-kilometre mark. You've gained just over 300 metres vertical from the lot and are now almost 1000 metres above sea level. Through the trees glimpses of the Tantalus Range peaks west across the Cheakamus Valley can be seen.

Another 20 minutes brings you to another white post—the 4-kilometre mark at 1120 metres elevation. Just after this point you may begin to think that Dante had it all wrong. His inferno spiralled endlessly downward into a pit of damnation, but a hiker's vision of hell is unending switchbacks up a steep, dry slope on a 30° C day.

Another 25 minutes should bring the next white post, marking 5 kilometres and 1280 metres vertical. Ten minutes farther are the first views of The Barrier.

This fascinating geological formation is essentially a big natural dam that formed about 12,000 years ago when lava pouring from an erupting Mount Price encountered a big

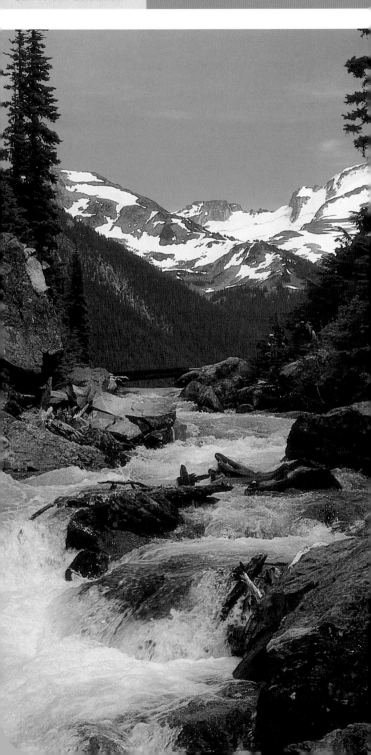

glacier. The precipitous cliff with its sharp-crested ridges and fractured face is actually the result of an 1855 landslide when a slab of rock about 500 metres long, 300 metres high and 500 metres deep sheared from The Barrier.

Mosey onward for another 10 minutes to the 6-kilometre marker at 1350 metres high. A few minutes distant is a major trail junction and the end of most of the vertical gain. To the left is Taylor Meadows and Black Tusk Meadows, but stay straight ahead to Garibaldi Lake, 3 kilometres distant.

> When The Barrier was formed, an estimated 45 million tonnes of rock snaked down one slope of Rubble Creek then up the other, knocking out huge swathes of forest, sweeping as far as the Cheakamus River, 5 kilometres distant, before coming to a dusty rest. Daisy Lake was then formed.

A level trail leads through the trees, emerging a few minutes later to an open view of The Barrier and the shores of Barrier Lake. After almost two hours on the trail, this is the place to splash some water on your face or soak your bandanna, but wait a little farther for a fast-flowing creek to refill your water bottle.

As the trail winds to the far end of Barrier Lake, it presents a stunning view of Tantalus Mountain framed in the saddle from where you emerged. A bit farther is the 7-kilometre marker at 1390 metres high. And just beyond that is Lesser Garibaldi Lake, its blue-green colour a hint to the cooler temperatures and glacial origins. Cross a wooden bridge over tumbling Taylor Creek.

Another 10 minutes brings you to a signpost noting a trail to Taylor Meadows. Another five minutes to the 8-kilometre marker at 1450 metres. And five more minutes brings you to yet another trail deviation to Taylor Meadows. (Continue straight to the lake.)

Soon, you'll cross the bridge over the creek that feeds from Garibaldi Lake to Lesser Garibaldi. Just a few hundred metres farther is the big lake itself—more than 5 kilometres long, 4 kilometres wide and 300 metres deep. In summer, the water is cool, not icy—perfect for a dip after a long hot hike.

If you're staying overnight, head for the campground 400 metres farther. If not, just find yourself a spot, explore the shore and Battleship Islands and take in the views of mountains, glaciers and lake, which made the area so entrancing that it was set aside as a provincial park in 1917.

Garibaldi Lake outlet.

46 PANORAMA RIDGE

Distance: 10 km (from Garibaldi Lake)	Rating: Moderate
	Season: July to October
Elevation gain: 630 m	Topographical map:
High point: 2100 m	Cheakamus River 92G/14
Time needed: 5 hours	Trail map: Page 211

Note: Dogs are not allowed in Garibaldi Provincial Park. For this hike, a topographical map and binoculars are highly recommended.

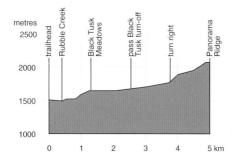

O UR HIKE STARTS FROM THE CAMP-ground at Garibaldi Lake, where sleeping alongside wow scenery means you'll have only 100 metres more elevation gain than if you were to start from the Taylor Meadows campground.

From Garibaldi Lake, cross the bridge over the outlet and ascend the switchbacks for about 15 to 20 minutes until you emerge onto the flowered flats of Black Tusk Meadows. Soon, the trail crosses a small creek, then reaches a junction. Taylor Campground is to the left, but we'll go right. Continue through the meadows.

In 1912, William Gray, a founding member of the BC Mountaineering Club (BCMC), bushwhacked, cleared and marked a route from the point where Rubble Creek meets the Cheakamus River to these meadows. The blaze marks are still visible on some trees, including the final marker, which bears Gray's words: 'Last blaze thank God the task is done.'

A short distance farther, the trail to Black Tusk bears off to the left. Continue straight ahead through the meadows. They offer magnificent views of Garibaldi Lake, Mount Price and other peaks of the park to the south. To the west are views of the glaciated spires and parapets of the Tantalus Range.

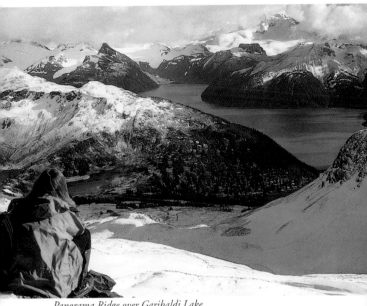

Panorama Ridge over Garibaldi Lake.

Thirty minutes of such happy wandering brings you to the junction with the Panorama Ridge Trail. The path straight ahead continues for another 11.5 kilometres through the Cinder Flats and Helm Valley to Cheakamus Lake. But we'll go right towards Black Tusk Lake, which is often ice-covered as late as July and August.

In 1912, Gray was also the man who introduced John Davidson, the first provincial botanist and later founder of the Vancouver Natural History Society, to the Black Tusk area. That year, Davidson and 10 BCMC members made the trek from Vancouver to the meadows by ferry, bus and foot, and set up camp. During the next 10 days, Davidson named many of the previously anonymous features, including Mimulus Lake, visible just west of Black Tusk Lake.

Follow the trail through scrubby heather meadows and occasional snowpatches and onto the flanks of the ridge ahead. From the ridge top is an expansive view of the Cinder flats and, in the near distance, Cinder Cone.

The eroded hill is what remains of one of the most recent eruptions in Garibaldi Park only a few centuries ago. It is, says geologist William Mathews, a product of 'explosive volcanism,' which hurled red-hot cinder bombs hundreds of metres from the main vent. Evidence of an even older volcanic cone can be seen tucked under Cinder Cone's western slope.

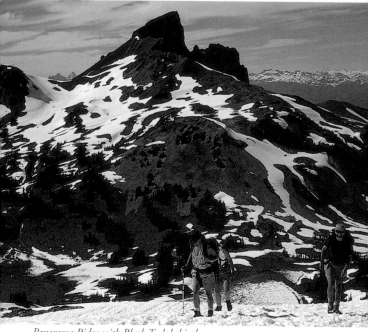

Panorama Ridge with Black Tusk behind.

Breathe deep and continue up along the rocky trail lined with red and white heather and the occasional mountain hemlock. When crossing rock scree, careful footwork is required. Follow the cairns and tracks in the snow up, up, up first to a false summit, then up a final scramble to the 2100-metre high point.

Here, the sweeping views make the origin of Panorama Ridge's name obvious. Directly north is a striking view of Black Tusk, sliding to the east is Helm Lake, Cinder Cone and the Helm Glacier spilling off nearby Gentian Peak. To the east is Castle Towers Mountain, Phyllis' Engine and Mount Carr, from which the Sphinx Glacier sweeps toward Garibaldi.

The ancient granite that makes up Empetrum Ridge, Castle Towers and the mountains above Sphinx Glacier was formed almost 200 million years ago. In those days, Garibaldi Park was sub-tropical lowland. Dinosaurs roamed its shallow valleys; the first small mammals struggled to survive.

But most of the features seen today are the result of two cataclysmic processes: volcanism and glaciation. Mount Garibaldi, to the south, is the remnant of a massive volcanic complex formed between 10,000 and 15,000 years ago. As vast glaciers receded north, the release of their weight on

The terrain is home to a species of lichen previously unknown in the region—*Tholurna dissimilis*, discovered in 1971 on the wind-scoured ridges of Cinder Cone, by UBC plant scientist George Otto. Lichens are remarkable little lifeforms. Native Peoples used them for years as an emergency food, as medicines to treat ailments such as pneumonia, and in dyes. Mountain goats, sheep and deer feed on them. Lichens are also extremely sensitive to air pollution, and so are good indicators of air quality.

the land triggered intense volcanic activity. Garibaldi, the volcano, belched thick clouds of ash and spewed burning rivers of lava.

An even older formation is visible high above the lake's south end: the flat-topped black monolith known as The Table. It's believed that about a million years ago, when great glaciers covered most of North America, The Table was formed by a volcano that erupted under the ice. With each eruption, hot lava melted out a channel higher and higher, but because of the pressure of the ice, the lava solidified in a block rather than the traditional cone shape.

Bring out your topographical map and binoculars; you could spend hours scanning the horizon while munching on a well-deserved lunch. Just leave enough time to get back to the campground in daylight.

47 BLACK TUSK

Distance: 14 km (from	Rating: Moderate
Garibaldi Lake)	Season: Late July to October
Elevation gain: 850 m	Topographical map:
High point: 2316 m	Brandywine Falls 92J/3
Time needed: 5 hours	Trail map: Page 211

Note: Dogs are not allowed in Garibaldi Provincial Park.

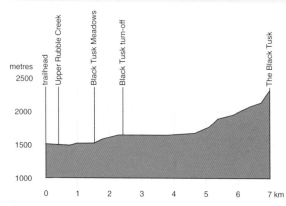

THE BLACK TUSK IS ONE OF THOSE UNMIS-takable landmarks that one seems to see from just about anywhere on the Squamish to Whistler corridor. Because of its ubiquitous presence, it looms large in the hearts and minds of valley-bound hikers.

As a dayhike from base camp at Garibaldi Lake or Taylor Meadows, Black Tusk is a perfect day of alpine meadows, a good aerobic workout and stunning mountain scenery. As a dayhike from the Black Tusk parking lot, it's a 32-kilometre, 10-hour long bad idea.

If you come from Taylor Meadows, the trip is a little easier and a kilometre shorter than if you come from Garibaldi Lake. For staying at the campground with the more superb scenery, lakeside folks have an extra 100 metres of elevation gain to hike.

From Garibaldi Lake, cross the bridge over the outlet creek and ascend steadily on switchback after switchback for about 15 to 20 minutes to emerge into subalpine, which marks the beginning of Black Tusk Meadows.

Soon, the trail crosses a small creek then reaches a junction. The Taylor Campground lies 2 kilometres to the left. But we'll go right, continuing through meadows that in summer are resplendent with wildflowers, and in autumn are ablaze with fall colours.

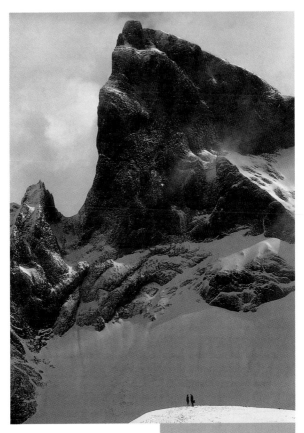

In the 1920s, '30s and '40s, Black Tusk Meadows was home to large camps each summer. Supplies were brought in by packhorse and the impact of all those horse hooves eventually wore a deep rut in the fragile meadow environment. To avoid the first rut, later packhorses followed a route parallel to the first and created a second rut. Much work has been done in subsequent years to restore the meadows. But a big part of it depends on conscientious hikers staying on the designated trails and off the meadows.

Gaze upon a place known to the Squamish people as 'Tak-tak-a-moh-yin-tla-ain-ain-ya-ha-an,' or 'The Landing Place of the Thunderbird.' Here on this ebony precipice, they believed, the supernatural creature lived. When it flapped its wings, thunder rolled across the land. When mortals ventured too close, lightning flashed from its eyes.

Five hundred metres past the junction, the trail to Black Tusk bears left. (Straight continues to the Panorama Ridge junction—see page 216—Cinder Flats, Helm Creek and Cheakamus Lake.) Steadily and seriously, the trail winds upward through more meadow, passing countless little streams along the way. Take as many water and breather breaks as you need, turning around occasionally to see the ever-expanding view as you gain more and more elevation.

Eventually, the trail leads from lush meadow to rocky talus and, an hour or so from the junction, arrives at a level shoulder well below the Tusk but with ample views and a ready excuse to stop for a break. If you've had enough for the day, this spot can be your lunch spot and turnaround point, replete with awesome views of Garibaldi Lake, Panorama Ridge and tiny Mimulus and Black Tusk lakes below, with other mountain features such as The Table, Sphinx Glacier and Mount Garibaldi farther distant.

From here, it's hard to imagine that there was once a time when these bluffs were once undersea. Remnant fossils are still found occasionally.

For those with more energy to burn, the route to the saddle east of the Tusk is a steep climb up, up, up. Fifteen to 20 minutes of slogging up rock and, in many months, snow brings you to a narrow saddle with big views east to Helm Valley, Cinder Cone and mountains beyond such as Corrie Peak and Mount Davidson.

If you have any discomfort with precipitous places, you'll be noticing it about now. Again, this can be your turnaround point, or you can follow the trail right along the ridge to a perfect perch for lunch. Or spend another 15 to 20 minutes of steep hiking to the base of the Black Tusk, well worth the effort just to see close-up what it is made of. What was once molten lava has crystallized into a mass of black rock columns compressed together. Millions of tiny crenellations betray the rock's brittle nature, and to be safe, hikers should go no further than here. Leave the points and heights farther distant to experienced climbers and mountaineers.

It is thought that the Black Tusk was one of the first geologically modern features to form in the Garibaldi area—an ancient volcano born 25 to 26 million years ago. As millennium after millennium passed, wind and weather wore away the softer ash and rock of its gentle slopes, leaving only the volcano's hard basalt core.

When you've finished absorbing the ancient wonder of the Tusk, retrace your steps to the base camp at Garibaldi Lake.

SEA TO SKY CORRIDOR

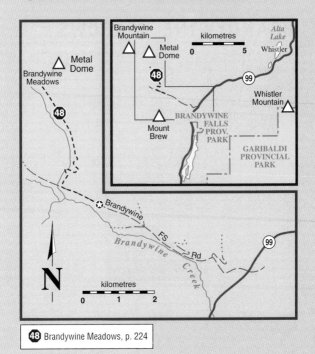

48 Brandywine Meadows, p. 224

48 BRANDYWINE MEADOWS

Distance: 6 km

Elevation gain: 500 m

High point: 1500 m

Time needed: 3–4 hours

Rating: Moderate

Season: July to October

Topographical map:
 Brandywine Falls 92J/3

Trail map: Page 223

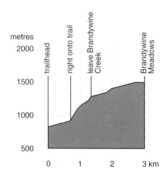

SOME HIKES GET STUCK IN YOUR BRAIN AS being particular to one season. Brandywine Meadows is one of them. And autumn is the season to hike it.

The sopping grounds of spring have passed, the bugs of summer are history, the temperatures are cooler and the fall colours are dazzling. About the only drawback is the fewer hours of daylight in which to enjoy one of the prettiest fall hikes in southwestern BC.

Even the drive to the trailhead is easy on the eyes. Head north on Highway 99 with its views of Howe Sound, the Squamish Chief, forests and peaks towards Brandywine Falls. About 3 kilometres past Brandywine Falls Provincial Park, you'll need to turn onto the Brandywine Forest Service Road. It's on the west side of the highway, where it is a double-lane section. Rather than attempt a life-threatening left turn from the fast lane in front of oncoming traffic, pull right off the road and wait for traffic to clear.

The logging road has some rugged, steep sections, as well as shallow ditches, and, if it's been raining, mud. Follow the road for about 4.5 kilometres to a three-way fork. Take the middle road and continue for another 2 kilometres.

If you've got a four-wheel drive vehicle, you can make it right to the trailhead proper. Otherwise, be prepared to walk a portion of the road, when you come to a section that your non-wilderness car can't handle.

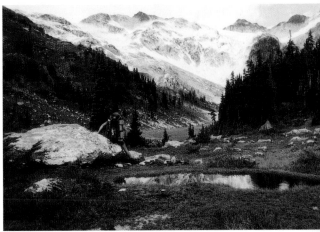

Brandywine Meadows.

Look for the brown Forest Service sign on the right side of the road for the start of the trail. From here, it's 500 metres of elevation gain and 3 kilometres of trail to the meadows.

The trail follows Brandywine Creek for the first few hundred metres. Later, near the top, the creek makes an appearance again nearer to its glacial source. (If you stop at the provincial park on the way home, you can see the same creek tumble down over Brandywine Falls on the last leg of its journey to Daisy Lake.)

The falls, the creek and the mountain got their name, it is said, in one of two ways. One version says that back in 1910 a surveyor and an axeman made a bet on the height of the falls. One man bet a bottle of wine, the other a bottle of brandy. The winner got the brandy and named the falls Brandywine.

The other version takes place in 1890, when two old-timers apparently passed out after lacing their tea too generously with brandy and wine. Which version is true is something to ponder while you hike on.

The trail turns from the creek and into the forest, where autumn brings a plethora of mushrooms sprouting through the damp humus of the ground.

What we call mushrooms are actually similar to the fruit of a tree, except in the case of the mushrooms, the tree is an often vast underground system of fungus. Mushrooms are how fungi proliferate. When the mushrooms ripen, they expel their seed contents to the elements—wind, water, animals—which then carry the budding baby fungi to a new nursery. And *voilà*, one day, a new fungal community.

Maybe you'll spot a scattering of *Cortinarius violaceous*—distinctive dark purple mushrooms, more commonly known as violet corts—or huge clusters of yellow sulphur tufts. Both types of mushrooms are beautiful, but quite deadly.

The forest here is dark and dense, but sunlight still streams through in places. If you're fortunate enough to catch the light early in the morning, while mist still wraps around the trees, you may see a phenomena I call 'mistflowers'—rosettes of rainbow-coloured light flowering around a tree trunk. As the light grows stronger, the 'flowers' grow bigger and more colourful.

After about an hour's worth of hiking through the forest, often boggy, sometimes muddy, finally there is light at the top of the trail. From here, the path scoots along the lower edge of a meadow, hopping up onto cross-hatched logs from time to time, to stay above the muck.

In 30 to 45 minutes, the trail rejoins Brandywine Creek and continues into a glacier-scoured hanging valley. In autumn, the meadows on both sides smoulder in hues of gold and ochre, scarlet and mauve. Fat, juicy blueberries are found in abundance here. As are bears. On my first fall trip to Brandywine Meadows, my hiking buddy and I spotted a black sow bear, along with two brown cubs, high on the west slope. It was a lovely sight...from a distance.

At the valley's end, the shoulder of Brandywine Mountain is visible, wrapped in a shimmering glacier. The true peak is just out of sight. It's possible to wander farther into the meadows. But if you do, don't stray from the trail. The tiny plants and shrubs that make up the meadows are extremely fragile; so is the thin soil beneath them. It takes a very long time—years, decades or more—for alpine meadows to recover from trampling and other human-generated disturbances.

So, eat your lunch, poke about and enjoy all the pleasures of an autumn day, responsibly. Then, leaving yourself a comfortable two hours of daylight to get back, head down the way you came.

WHISTLER AREA

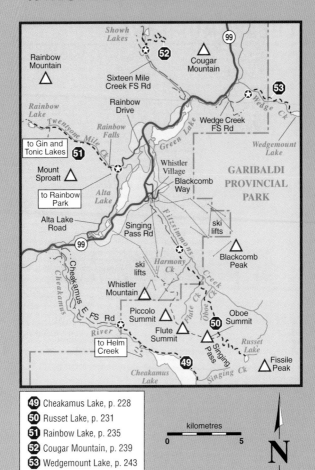

Rainbow Mountain ▲

Showh Lakes

99

Cougar Mountain ▲

53

Wedge Ck

Sixteen Mile Creek FS Rd

52

Rainbow Drive

Rainbow Lake

Rainbow Falls

Twentyone Mile Ck

Green Lake

Wedge Creek FS Rd

Wedgemount Lake

to Gin and Tonic Lakes 51

Rainbow Ck

GARIBALDI PROVINCIAL PARK

Mount Sproatt ▲

to Rainbow Park

Alta Lake

Whistler Village

Blackcomb Way

Alta Lake Road

99

Singing Pass Rd

Fitzsimmons Creek

ski lifts

Cheakamus

Cheakamus E FS Rd

ski lifts

Harmony Ck

Blackcomb Peak ▲

Whistler Mountain ▲

Piccolo Summit ▲

Flute Ck

Oboe Creek

Oboe Summit ▲

50

River

to Helm Creek

Flute Summit ▲

Singing Pass

Russet Lake

49

Cheakamus Lake

Singing Ck

Fissile Peak ▲

49 Cheakamus Lake, p. 228
50 Russet Lake, p. 231
51 Rainbow Lake, p. 235
52 Cougar Mountain, p. 239
53 Wedgemount Lake, p. 243

kilometres
0   5

N

49 CHEAKAMUS LAKE

Distance: 14 km	Season: May to November
Elevation gain: Minimal	Topographical map:
High point: 915 m	Whistler 92J/2
Time needed: 5 hours	Trail map: Page 227
Rating: Easy	Note: Dogs are not allowed on the trail.

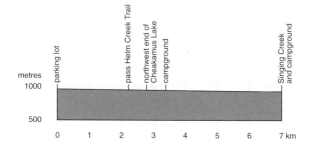

FED BY CONSTANT MELTWATER FROM THE glaciers of Garibaldi Provincial Park, Cheakamus Lake seems like the perfect hiking destination for any blisteringly hot day. And yes, the waters are refreshing, but the best time for a long amble along the lake's northern shore is autumn.

Although higher alpine destinations can require layers of clothing against the cold, at Cheakamus' 900-metre elevation the air is merely cool and filled with the scent of withering leaves. The crowds of summer have returned home. With daylight hours dwindling, the hike is long enough to feel like a satisfied day's outing, not a hurried summer leftover.

To get to the trailhead, follow Highway 99 towards Whistler. Then, just as you near the mountain municipality's southern boundary, watch for the provincial park signs pointing the way to Cheakamus Lake and turn right, onto Cheakamus Lake Road.

After 200 metres or so of pavement, veer left onto the Cheakamus Lake Forest Service Road and follow it for about 6 kilometres to the trailhead. Along the way are markers noting stops of interest on a forestry tour, but you'll know you've reached your destination when you see the familiar green BC Parks outhouse and parked cars.

At the trailhead, a sign shows the whole of Garibaldi Provincial Park, in which Cheakamus Lake sits. There may also be a notice of bears in the area. Although bears usually

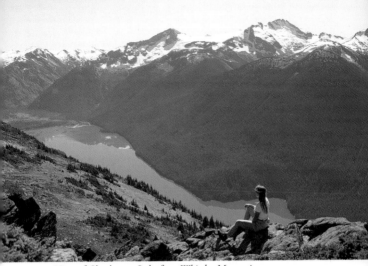

View of Cheakamus Lake from Whistler Mountain.

keep to themselves, it's still a good idea to make noise—sing, talk, whistle—when on the trail, just to alert them to your presence and give them opportunity to move to a distance more comfortable for you and the bears.

Leaving the parking lot behind, the trail meanders through boulder field and slide alder for the first 10 minutes or so, then slips into the forest where the air is cool, lush and scented with balsam. The deeper you get, the bigger the cedar, fir and hemlock seem to grow.

After 30 minutes of forested bliss, you'll come to an intersection with the Helm Creek Trail, which heads southwest across the Cheakamus River along Helm Creek towards Black Tusk Meadows and Garibaldi Lake. Save that trip for a longer summer day and continue straight ahead.

By this time, you'll likely have noticed that mountain bikers use the trail too. Most are courteous and give way to hikers, as they should, but it's best to stay alert.

Cheakamus Lake really is a multi-use destination. I've seen people portage a canoe along the trail to the lakeshore, and quite a few fellow hikers come with fishing gear in hand to try their luck with the rainbow trout and Dolly Varden char resident in the lake's icy waters.

Soon, the Cheakamus River, which you've heard since leaving the lot, will come into view. Soon after, the lake appears— a turquoise jewel ringed by emerald forests and diamantine peaks.

The trail continues alongside the big trees and big views, occasionally passing through areas crowded in summer with wildflowers such as ruby-hued Indian paintbrush, sapphire-coloured lupines and golden tiger lilies.

In fall, equally colourful groupings of mushrooms, toadstools and fungus can be found.

Years ago, an old trapper's cabin squatted on this spot. Now all that remains are a few trees cut with square notches used to keep marten traps from freezing. Another cabin not much farther away was still standing as recently as 1971. But it also is no more.

A sign notes the 3-kilo-metre mark and another BC Parks map to help pick out the names of the surrounding mountains—Corrie Peak, Castle Towers Mountain and Mount Davidson. The latter summit is named after John Davidson, who in 1911 was appointed to conduct the first botanical survey of BC. He also started a collection that would eventually become the University of British Columbia Botanical Garden. (While the UBC campus was being built, Davidson convinced the province to set aside 0.8 hectares of land at Colony Farm in Port Coquitlam. Thus was born Canada's first-ever botanical garden.)

In 1912, Davidson joined a BC Mountaineering Club trip to the Garibaldi area. He conducted topographical, geological and botanical research in the area, named features such as Mimulus and Parnassus Creek, and spearheaded efforts to have the area set aside as a provincial park.

The trail follows the lakeside, and it's worth a stop to take in some of the remarkable features that were formally protected as parkland in 1927, and to dip trail-warmed toes into the glacier-fed lake.

After an hour or so, through forest, along gravel beaches and across tiny streams, is the end of the trail near Singing Creek, 7 kilometres from where you started.

Stroll down to the alluvial gravel fan at lakeside, find the perfect spot to listen to the siren song of the tinkling creek, to drink in the views, soak your toes and break for a long, leisurely lunch. Then, when you're ready, retrace your steps to the start.

RUSSET LAKE

Distance: 29 km	Rating: Strenuous
Elevation gain: 1250 m	Season: July to October
High point: 2000 m	Topographical map:
Time needed: 10 hours	Whistler 92J/2
	Trail map: Page 227

Note: Dogs are not allowed in Garibaldi Provincial Park.

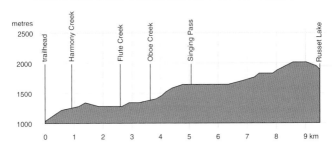

T HE TRIP TO RUSSET LAKE HAS ALWAYS BEEN stiff, but recent access changes make it even stiffer. Still, it's worth the effort. Among the rewards to be reaped are moss-covered forest, fragile alpine meadows and stunning mountain views. And you can always turn around at Singing Pass (making for a 20-kilometre, 7- to 8-hour roundtrip) instead of continuing farther to Russet.

To get to the trailhead, head north on Highway 99 to Whistler. At Village Gate Boulevard, turn right and head to the T-junction at Blackcomb Way. Turn right again. About 300 metres distant is a bus loop—and where you'll start on foot once you've parked your vehicle.

From the bus loop, head up the gravel road for about 5 kilometres to reach what was, until recently, the parking area and true trailhead.

Even here, the views are great. Blackcomb Mountain towers across the same valley through which the icy green Fitzsimmons Creek tumbles. In autumn, a pastiche of crimson, russet and gold autumn foliage paints the mountainside.

Squirrels chatter and scold from nearby branches. Steller's (shown) and gray jays flit from tree to tree.

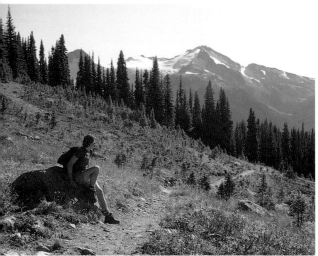

Singing Pass, en route to Russet Lake.

From the signboard, the trail starts narrow and leads southeast. For the next 2.5 to 3 hours, the trail leads steadily uphill through the forested mountainside. So pace yourself and get a good conversation going—discuss the nature of the universe, the future of the planet, the inexplicable appeal of old *Star Trek* episodes that you've already seen 15 or 20 times.

Not far from the start, the trail passes the entrance to an old mine shaft. Twisted, rusting metal track careens off the cliff. Mining activity began in the Whistler area in 1910. In the area above Fitzsimmons Creek were Green Lake Mining and Milling Company claims with names such as Iron Wedge, Eldorado, Hard Cash and Midget. Tunnels were blasted and drilled through low-grade ore showing traces of gold, silver and copper. There was never quite enough to turn a profit.

Continue along the trail that was first built as a government pack trail about 1900. Soon, Harmony Creek can be heard tinkling in the distance. And then, before you know it, you'll find yourself boulder-hopping across.

Winding steadily upward, the trail passes the 2-kilometre marker, then Flute Creek, then the 3-kilometre marker.

Soon, you reach a sign noting the boundary of Garibaldi Provincial Park. If you've ridden a bike from the village, the road ends here for your bicycle. Take the left fork (right goes to the base of the blue chair on Whistler Mountain).

Trundle steadily upward through the cool of the forest past the 3-kilometre marker. Just beyond is a good viewpoint of

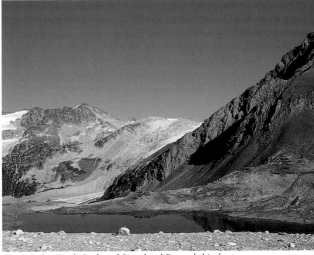

Russet Lake, Fissile Peak and Spearhead Range behind.

Blackcomb Mountain created a few years ago by a windstorm that blew down quite a few of the surrounding tall trees. Not much farther is Oboe Creek. If you haven't yet taken a water or rest break, do so here.

Then it's back to the trail and the continuing low-gear grunt. Another 15 minutes should bring you to the 4-kilometre marker. Just beyond, an old trail built by Whistler pioneer Bill Bailiff branches downhill to Melody Creek. (That trail is usually wet and not really worth taking as an alternative to the well-constructed path on which you're already walking. Think of it more as a point of interest.) Bailiff, who came to the Whistler area in 1913 as a worker with the Pacific Great Eastern Railway, maintained a trapline in this area.

Another 30 minutes or so brings you to Melody Creek and subalpine meadows. The trees are sparser and shorter. The understorey changes to damp meadow, the perfect medium for moisture-loving wildflowers such as western anemones and marsh marigolds.

The long hike up can sometimes feel a little claustrophobic on sunny days, but now you're in the open and not too far from Singing Pass. Within 15 minutes, the trail passes the junction with the Musical Bumps Trail over Oboe, flute and Piccolo Summits to the Whistler gondola. (This hike is usually overrun with crowds and is best left for another day.)

Soon, wildflowers begin to appear along the trail—delicate yellow glacier lilies, scarlet Indian paintbrush and deep blue lupines among others. Late June to early August is the best time for this flower show, but it depends to a large extent on how much snow fell the previous winter and how fast the snow is melting.

In autumn, the blooms are gone, but the warm, muted colours of heather and blueberry bush mingled with fewer folks on the trail create an equally inviting atmosphere.

By the time you reach the summit of Singing Pass, you'll probably feel like singing yourself. This, however, is not the origin of the name. The name Singing Pass came from Ottar Brandvold, one of the trio who built Diamond Head Lodge farther south in Garibaldi Park. He was inspired during a camping trip in the 1950s, when he heard the wind singing over the slopes.

With Russet Lake still another 40 minutes and 2.5 kilometres distant, it's worth stopping here for a good rest, some water and a snack.

Then regain the trail as it heads left up the east side of a knoll. After a couple of zigs and zags, the trail meanders through a veritable moonscape of talus and scree with outstanding views of distant summits such as Corrie Peak, Mount Davidson and Castle Towers Mountain.

Soon, the trail drops to Russet Lake. Take a long and well-deserved rest at lakeside with the massive Fissile Peak above—and below, reflected in the lake waters. Gaze northeast to the peaks and glaciers of the Spearhead Range. Breathe deep. Eat lunch. Poke your head in the BC Mountaineering Club cabin.

After absorbing enough alpine ambiance, retrace all your steps. After the push out of Russet, it's virtually all downhill.

RAINBOW LAKE 51

Distance: 16 km	Rating: Moderate
Elevation gain: 850 m	Season: July to October
High point: 1470 m	Topographical maps:
Time needed: 6 hours	Whistler 92J/2 and
(allow more if snow	Brandywine 92J/3
is on the trail)	Trail map: Page 227

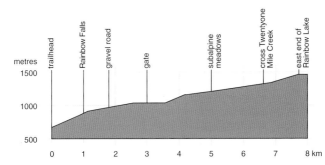

RAINBOW LAKE, NEAR WHISTLER, CAN BE the perfect summer hiking destination. The only thing you need to consider is snow depth. Although it may be blazing hot in the valley, snow regularly hangs around near Rainbow well into July.

To get to the trailhead, follow Highway 99 north towards Whistler. After crossing the railway tracks and passing Function Junction (at Alpha Lake Road), turn left onto Alta Lake Road and drive high above the west side of Alta Lake for about 7 kilometres.

Just after the sign for Rainbow Park on the right, is the sign for the Rainbow Trail on the left. Park here at the mouth of Twentyone Mile Creek.

The trail starts on the south side of the creek (that would be your left if you're looking upstream). Follow it up through the trees for a couple of hundred metres to where the trail forks. Bear right, staying along the creek.

A few minutes brings you to a sign for Rainbow Falls. Go right for a short side-trip worth every step of a short uphill section. Taking this route also lets you escape the heat of a summer day by staying in the trees instead of trudging along a dusty hot gravel road.

Less than 15 minutes from the trailhead, you'll come to the falls. Clouds of mist rise from the plunging creek waters. If the

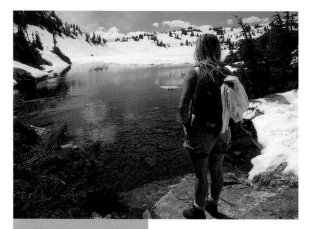

A tumble of falls is only minutes up the trail, followed by wildflowers and subalpine views and ending with the large alpine lake, set in a scenic mountain bowl.

wind is right, the mist will blow a refreshing spray in your direction. If the light is right, you might see a rainbow.

The falls are actually a succession of precipitous tiers, the water boiling and churning through cauldron after cauldron of rock. If you do explore farther than the uppermost falls, be extremely careful near the cliff edges or you could give the falls a second meaning.

Rainbow Falls has been a popular destination for Whistler-area hikers, even before the place was known as Whistler. In 1914, Alex and Myrtle Philip built the Rainbow Lodge on Alta Lake; within a few years it was the most popular resort west of Jasper.

Hikers would head for Rainbow Falls and points distant along trails lined with old-growth. But in 1951, despite the appeals of local residents and the ratepayer association, the surrounding forest was logged. The subsequent slash fire got out of control and for three weeks, a fire burned—all the way to the bluffs of Sproatt Mountain.

After viewing the falls, regain the trail and follow it right, as indicated by the Rainbow Lake sign. In 10 to 15 minutes, the trail emerges to the gravel road right next to a water supply building.

Turn and look across the Whistler valley for views of Wedge, Blackcomb and Whistler mountains, the latter two criss-crossed with ski runs. Much of Blackcomb was actually logged in the

1940s. Loggers would haul the trees off the hillside and into Lost Lake to be milled for lumber. Whistler Mountain wasn't logged until the mid-1960s in its preparation as a ski resort.

Follow the trail south as yet another sign indicates. At first, clusters of lupines dot the open road. Later, as the roadside foliage thickens, columbines, rosy twisted-stalk, bunchberry and goat's beard intermix with occasional glimpses of the mountains opposite.

Eventually, the road winds to an end at a gate. Those steel-thighed folk who have ridden a mountain bike thus far can lock it to the bike rack provided. From here on the trail is for feet only.

Although the trail switches back and forth, gaining in elevation, you can be thankful for the shady respite of the deepening forest. About 30 minutes in is a glade of sweet-smelling cedar and Douglas fir. And not much further, you'll cross a tributary of Twentyone Mile Creek on a two-log bridge. (Be careful, it can be slippery when wet.)

The forest is cool here as you wander under the coniferous canopy. Boardwalk and log bridges help negotiate the marshier sections, some with space-alien-sized skunk cabbage. Another 30 minutes brings another creek to cross. And, moments later, another creek spills down in a ribbon of falls, having originated at Gin and Tonic Lakes.

As you reach the 5-kilometre marker, just where the trail skirts the lower edges of a slide area, the trail emerges up and out of the forest and into subalpine meadows with their twisted, stunted cedar and yew trees and emerging views of Rainbow Mountain.

When still in the throes of spring run-off, the meadows can at times resemble weedy wading pools. Worry not, there is boardwalk to protect both your feet from the wet and the fragile meadow plants from your feet.

For the next 20 minutes, the trail gains some elevation as it winds back toward Twentyone Mile Creek. A perfectly placed bench just before the creek crossing makes for a good rest stop with wide-open views of the valley through which you've travelled.

The stout cable bridge that crosses the creek has its deckboards taken up every autumn. If you arrive before the deckboards are replaced in spring, you'll have to cross farther downstream.

Fifteen to 20 minutes of hiking brings another creek, which can be fast-slowing during the freshets. Crossing it may involve treading some makeshift bridges, such as the broken

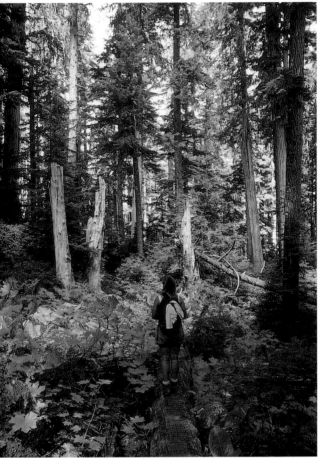

The Rainbow Lake Trail.

beam encountered on one trip, tricky both for balance and for slipperiness. Take your time and use whatever handholds are available.

How long it takes to make the final push upward will depend on the presence or depth of snow. If the trail is clear, 10 or 15 minutes will bring you to the lake. Figure about twice as much time in snow-covered conditions.

Soon, though, Rainbow Lake makes its appearance, snuggled between Rainbow Mountain to the north and Sproatt Ridge to the south, and the pass overlooking the Pemberton Icecap at the far end of the tarn. Find a dry rock to sit on while you slather on some sunscreen and eat your well-deserved lunch.

And, after a restful repose, return the way you came.

COUGAR MOUNTAIN 52

Distance: 6 km	Rating: Easy
Elevation gain: 150 m	Season: May to October
High point: 1065 m	Topographical map:
Time needed: 2 hours	Whistler 92J/2
	Trail map: Page 227

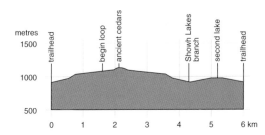

EARLY IN THE 1900S, BEFORE SKI RESORTS, high-end shopping malls and expensive real estate defined Whistler, it was a sleepy retreat from big city living.

The first settlers arrived early in the 20th century and, not long after, the first Pacific Great Eastern train pulled into town. Some of those early trains brought people with a financial interest in the timber that covered valleys and slopes. In 1926, the first mill was built on Green Lake; by the 1930s, other smaller sawmills dotted other lakeshores.

That's why it's hard to find much old-growth in the Whistler area. Fortunately, there is a lush exception: the ancient cedars of Cougar Mountain.

To get to the trailhead, follow Highway 99 to Whistler. Nine kilometres past Whistler Village, just after Green Lake comes to an end is the Sixteenmile Creek Forest Service Road. Watching carefully for oncoming traffic, turn left across the highway and onto the logging road. Stay right at the fork a few hundred metres distant. And at the next fork, 4 kilometres from the highway, stay right. (Left goes on the Tour du Soo, a killer 40-kilometre mountain bike ride on logging road and singletrack.)

One kilometre more brings you to a third fork. Go left to a parking area with a signboard and map, and park.

A narrow path just right of the signboard leads to an old spur road that will take you part of the way to Cougar Mountain. Note that on this multi-use trail you may encounter mountain bikes and ATVs.

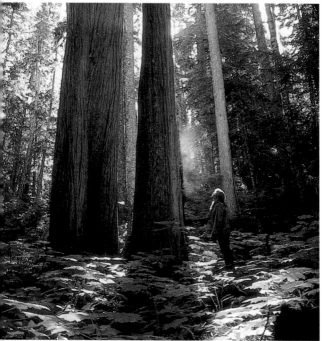

Ancient cedar grove, Cougar Mountain.

The brush here grows higher each year, but you do get occasional glimpses of Showh Lakes below and old cutblocks all around as you follow the rocky road up. The last bit of wide road is a short, steepish section of loose rocks. A newer side-trail just to the right is less steep and less rocky, so take your pick.

Where the trail makes its first hairpin turn to the left, look downslope to see a sweet water-lilied pond at the bottom of an ancient rockfall. As you continue up, there are more views of logged valleys and slopes. Some cuts are regenerating, and others are freshly cut.

Trees first began to be cut in the Whistler area with the arrival of settlers in the 1910s. But it wasn't until 1926, with the construction of the first mill, that the logging industry really got going.

Logging still goes on in the Whistler area, albeit more conscientiously and under better regulations. But it'll take a long, long time before groves such as the one ahead are seen again in this neck of the woods.

Where the trail proper begins, you can tell—not only by the height and girth of the trees, but by the sunbleached snags and witch's hair lichen that drips from tree limbs—that the forest

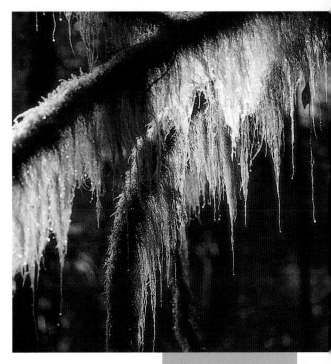

you're entering is older than the one you've just come through.

The trail passes over a rock outcrop piled with tiny cairns of gravity-defying stones. Fifty metres farther, a side-trail branches left to a view of Showh Lakes with Sisqa, Semam and Kwtamts peaks in the distance. The lookout makes a good spot for a water break or lunch.

Lichens are very slow-growing organisms, on average growing about 1 millimetre a year. They're also very old, some as much as 4000 years. Some are found almost exclusively in old-growth and provide needed components to the soil for a tree's continued growth.

After retracing your steps to the main trail, follow it downhill to a wooden bridge and across a tiny nameless creek. (Just before the bridge, on the right, is the trail on which you'll return.) The damp hollow you're now entering is the perfect medium for such moisture-loving species as skunk cabbage, devil's club and western red cedar.

Where blowdown has set up a Douglas fir just waiting to crash down on the trail, the big trees begin. Slim, stately cedars give way to larger and larger trees—many more than 60 metres high and almost 10 metres around. The trees are estimated to be 600 to 1000 years old.

For many people, western red cedar is the tree that defines British Columbia. It was used by Native Peoples for shelter, clothing, tools and transportation. Few cedars were actually felled before the arrival of non-Native people. Natives used fallen trees or boards split from standing trees (thus the term 'culturally modified trees').

According to Hilary Stewart in *Cedar: Tree of Life,* the power of the red cedar tree was said to be so strong a person could receive strength by standing with his or her back to the tree.

A Coast Salish myth says the Great Spirit created red cedar in honour of a man who was always helping others. Where such a man was buried, notes Stewart, a cedar tree would grow and continue to help others by providing roots for baskets, bark for clothing and wood for shelter.

After you enjoy this haven of old-growth and strength, follow the trail over a couple of small wooden bridges and a bit of rockfall to emerge at the creek and the first bridge. From there, it's almost all downhill to the logging road.

Before heading back to Whistler or points farther south, it's worth making the 30-minute side-trip to Showh Lakes, which you saw earlier from above.

WEDGEMOUNT LAKE 53

Distance: 14 km   Rating: Strenuous

Elevation gain: 1200 m   Season: July to September

High point: 1910 m   Topographical map:

Time needed: 7–8 hours   Whistler 92J/2

                                  Trail map: Page 227

Note: Dogs are not allowed in Garibaldi Provincial Park.

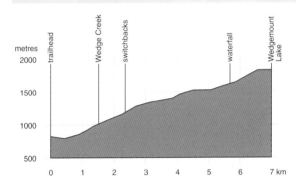

T HE HIKE TO WEDGEMOUNT LAKE IS THE high end of the hiking scale—in more ways than one. It features some of the most superb alpine scenery in the region—a turquoise lake, rugged granite peaks, diamantine glaciers—but it's also the toughest and the steepest hike in this book.

Although the hike to The Lions may have more vertical gain, it's also spread over a slightly longer distance. On the trail to The Lions, you'll climb 162.5 metres of vertical for every kilometre you hike. On the trail to Wedgemount Lake, every kilometre is 171.5 metres of vertical gain.

The steepest part of the trail to Wedgemount is also the highest portion. Thus, snow can linger well into summer, making for an unnerving ascent. For that reason and all the others, August is the optimum month for a hike. Think of July and September as weather-dependent.

To get to the trailhead, follow Highway 99 to Whistler. About 12 kilometres north of Whistler Village, follow the blue BC Parks sign right, across the railway tracks and over a small bridge. Turn left, then right, then left, and continue along a narrow road to the parking lot.

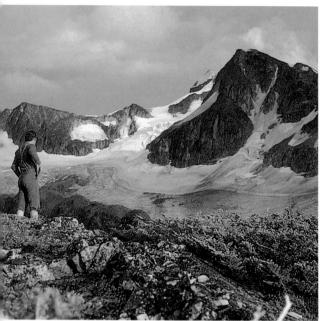

Wedgemount Lake Trail.

From here, the trail climbs gradually but steadily through second-growth forest. Before tourism, ski hills and glitzy shops, the lumber industry was the mainstay of Whistler. In fact, the first sawmill in the area was built by the three Barr brothers not far away—on the northeast shores of Green Lake in 1926. A few years later, the mill changed hands, then it burned to the ground. Another mill was built, and it operated until the mid-1950s.

Much of Whistler's low-elevation old-growth forests passed through the mill. One of the few remaining groves is just across the valley at Cougar Mountain (see page 239).

After 20 to 30 minutes, the trail meets Wedge Creek. For the next 2 to 2.5 hours, water is virtually nonexistent, so fill water bottles and soak bandannas here. Once across the creek, the trail switches back and continues upward. After passing one rockslide then another, the trail teasingly levels. Within seconds, however, it takes a sharp left and begins climbing again.

The good news is that you've come about halfway. The bad news is that the trail seems only to grow steeper the higher you go. This part of the hike is where it is helpful to find a mental task with which to occupy your mind for an hour or so. Figure

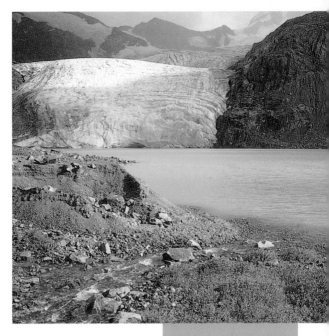

out the beginning of that great Canadian novel you've always wanted to write. Sketch out next year's Christmas card list. Or consider the tale of Whistler pioneer Charlie Chandler.

In the early 1900s, Chandler traded Wisconsin for the wilds of Whistler in an attempt to deal with a drinking problem. The solution, he figured, was to get away to the woods, some place where liquor wouldn't be handy.

In winter, Chandler ran a trapline on Wedge Creek as far as the pass, then a couple of kilometres down Billy Goat Creek on the Lillooet side. In summer he did odd jobs. But after getting some cash together, he'd head for town, live it up, then head home broke.

As recently as the 1980s, Wedge Glacier poured directly into the lake, occasionally calving a tiny herd of impossibly blue bergy bits. But global warming, with its warmer summers and sparser winter snowfall, has shrunk glaciers all over the world, and it has also caused the Wedge Glacier to retreat farther and farther upslope. Since 1850, it's estimated that the glacier has retreated about 1.5 kilometres.

In the winter of 1946, Chandler was found completely frozen, seated in a chair on his porch. His icy corpse, still seated, was transported to Rainbow Station and put on the train south.

Back on the hiking trail, your eyes will finally light on a waterfall that plunges more than 300 metres and seems all the more beautiful simply because of all the effort you've spent getting there. Rest, recover and contemplate the moment; the steepest is yet to come.

From here, the trail seems to rise almost vertically above the treeline and through scree slopes until finally, 30 minutes later, you top out. A 5 to 10-minute scamper is all that lies between you and the BC Mountaineering Club cabin. From there, it's a short scramble to the lakeshore.

At the lake's southeastern edge, the Wedge Glacier nestles near the shore. Although it is possible to wander the lakeshore to the glacier's snout, it is definitely not a good idea to wander either on top of the ice or inside the crevasses. Leave that to experienced mountaineers, who use the glacier as access to Wedge Mountain, the highest peak in Garibaldi Provincial Park.

Your way is also now all downhill, and be sure to allow almost the same amount of time to get down as you did to get up. The downward path is steep and the footing is occasionally tricky.

PEMBERTON AREA

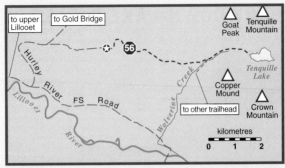

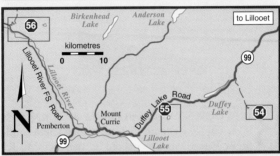

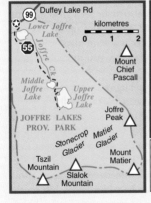

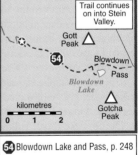

54 Blowdown Lake and Pass, p. 248
55 Joffre Lakes, p. 252
56 Tenquille Lake, p. 256

54 BLOWDOWN LAKE & PASS

Distance: 8 km	Rating: Moderate
Elevation gain: 600 m	Season: July to September
High point: 2100 m	Topographical map:
Time needed: 5 hours	Duffey Lake 92J/8
	Trail map: Page 247

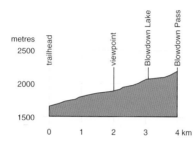

BLOWDOWN PASS IS PROBABLY BEST KNOWN as an easy-access route via Cottonwood Creek to the Stein Valley, now protected as the Stein Valley Heritage Park.

But the pass area and the lake also make for a great day-trip destination: there are good views and lots of optional alpine scrambles. In fact, Blowdown Lake is a good place to set up a weekend base camp, the better to allow you to explore more on the other side of the divide.

To get to the trailhead, head up Highway 99 to Pemberton. At the T-junction, zero your odometer and turn right, following the road to Mount Currie and the turnoff at 6.7 kilometres for the Duffey Lake Road. Follow the road as it passes through the St'atlimx Reserve, then along the shores of Lillooet Lake and up, up, up to Cayoosh Pass. Continue past Joffre Lakes Provincial Park until, about 56 kilometres from Pemberton, you see a yellow and black avalanche-control gate. Just on the other side is the Blowdown Creek logging road. Turn right and head uphill. Soon the road levels out and, 9 kilometres farther, comes to an open area where there is an old rusting wood and metal platform. This is the starting point for your hike.

For the first 10 to 15 minutes, walk up along the left fork of the road through alder saplings, fireweed and tiny spruce trees. The way then opens for 5 to 10 minutes' worth of views of the peaks to the west before the vegetation closes in again.

Where the road levels, there are great views southwest to an unnamed peak. And straight ahead are great views of another

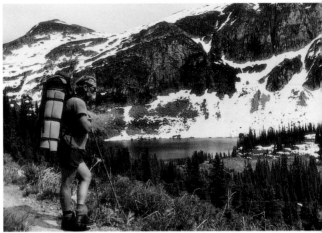

Blowdown Lake.

unnamed peak, this one with a star-shaped fan of scree. As the road climbs steadily uphill, it gradually enters second-growth forest. And after about 40 to 50 minutes of consistent huffing and puffing, there is a viewpoint and some rocks on which to sit for a water break.

The next section of road is definitely not the most scenic, but if you can luxuriate in just being outdoors and away from it all, the next 35 to 40 minutes should go quickly enough. You may also have the added distraction of seeing 4x4 vehicles parked on the roadside where they could not navigate a couple of nasty washouts.

Eventually, though, the road levels out. Soon another old road branches to the right and Blowdown Lake. If you're setting up camp or just want to stop for lunch before hitting the pass, it's only a 10-minute saunter to the lakeshore.

When you're ready to head for Blowdown Pass, retrace your steps to the main road and follow it as it bends into the trees

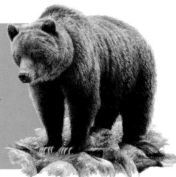

Grizzly bears frequent the area at certain times of the year, notably early summer. Make lots of noise on the road. And, if you're camping, be sure to hang your food and take all the usual precautions. See page 21 for more details.

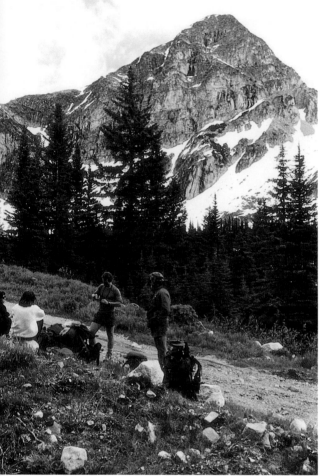

Along the trail.

then switches back. Within a few minutes, the lake reappears, shimmering beneath bluffs that are still snow-covered in July and August.

As you continue up the road, the trees get smaller and sparser. You've entered the 'AT zone,' or as it's more formally known, the Alpine Tundra biogeoclimatic zone. In parts farther south or west, the zone starts at around the 2250-metre mark. But here, in the transition zone between coastal and interior terrain, the AT zone starts as low as 1620 metres.

As with most alpine tundra areas, vegetation is pretty sparse, usually limited to hardier lichens, shrubs and trees that can endure the constant cold, wind and snow—sometimes even at the height of summer. (On one Canada Day weekend here, I awoke to ankle-deep snow that had fallen overnight.)

About 30 minutes or so from the lake, the road makes one final switchback and emerges to the summit of Blowdown Pass. From here, views stretch into the Cottonwood Creek Valley and beyond to Siwhe and Evenglow Mountains beyond.

The road actually continues farther into the Stein Park, although it is soon impassable unless on foot. The road was built earlier in the 20th century as access to the Silver Queen Mine, which apparently never really brought out any ore of any substance.

The peak immediately to the left is Gott Peak. It and nearby Gott Creek are named after Frank Gott, a Lillooet hunter, guide, rancher and prospector who managed to get into the 102nd Battalion to serve in World War I by dyeing his silver locks black. But despite his sharpshooting skills, he was sent back to Canada in 1917, as overage. Fifteen years later, he got into a feud with a game warden. When the warden tried to arrest him for possessing an untagged deer, Gott shot him in the back. The authorities eventually caught up with Gott and demanded his surrender.

'I am a soldier and I never surrender,' Gott reportedly replied. An officer opened fire, wounding Gott in the leg. He later died in hospital in Lytton, although it is said to be more from advanced tuberculosis, exposure and lack of nourishment than from the leg wound. Wardens and police officers aside, the public was in fact rather fond of Gott. He was given a military funeral. And a mountain.

The peak directly on the right is called either Gotcha Peak or Not Gott, depending on which wag you've asked. Either summit is easily achievable after a good bout of scrambling, and both have stunning views. Just be sure to watch your footing on the loose rock and the bluff edges and to leave enough time to return along the same route to camp or your vehicle within daylight.

55 JOFFRE LAKES

Distance: 11 km	Rating: Moderate
Elevation gain: 400 m	Season: Mid-July to mid-September
High point: 1600 m	Topographical map:
Time needed: 5 hours	Duffey Lake 92J/8
	Trail map: Page 247

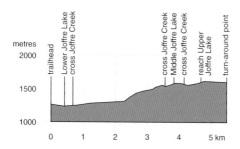

EVERY YEAR, THOUSANDS OF SUMMER visitors flock to the resort burg of Whistler. Some meander the low-elevation trails of Lost Lake, others head for an all-day outing at Rainbow Lake or Singing Pass. But unbeknownst to many people is one of the most gorgeous hikes that southwestern BC has to offer—a mere hour's drive north of Whistler.

Climbers have known about the Joffre area for years. For neophyte mountaineers, it's a wealth of easily accessed opportunities for gaining skills. For experienced climbers, there's glaciers to travel, peaks to summit and challenges galore.

Hikers took a little longer to discover Joffre's delights. And although the trails are busier now than they've ever been, it's still nothing compared to a backcountry Sunday afternoon at Whistler.

To get to the trailhead, follow Highway 99 to Pemberton, then bear right to Mount Currie. From here, follow the Duffey Lake Road for about 20 kilometres as it winds first through the St'atlimx Indian reserve, past Lillooet Lake and steadily upward towards Cayoosh Pass. Then just watch for the familiar provincial park signs for Joffre.

Joffre Lakes was first created as a recreational area, but in 1995 it gained full provincial park status.

From the parking lot, the trail takes only moments to reach views of the lowest of Joffre's three lakes. A short side-trail leads to a viewpoint of the lake, but you'll see similar views by following the signposted way to Upper Joffre.

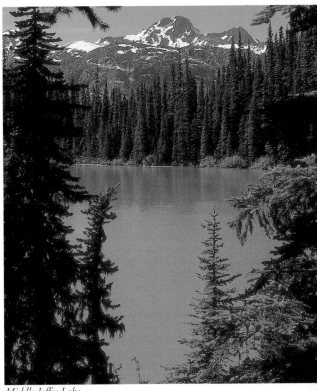

Middle Joffre Lake.

A compact gravel path travels high above a bug-infested marsh, across a small wooden bridge across Lower Joffre Creek and into old-growth forest. At this elevation and latitude, the forest is mostly hemlock and spruce—big trees for this neck of the woods. The most abundant fauna are the bugs: mosquitoes, blackflies and other tiny annoyances. Take insect repellent.

The gravel path eventually cedes to dirt trail and climbs gradually upward, occasionally crossing a tiny feeder stream. About 25 minutes in, the trail forks. Stay left, on the lower trail. (Right is the old trail, now overgrown and disused.) The trail descends a steepish section then levels off into a boulder field. At first, you're shaded from the heat of a summer's day by the alder, shrubs and other greenery.

> The forest floor is lush with the dogwood-like flowers of bunchberry, the tiny white sprays of foamflower and the big, ubiquitous and best avoided specimens of devil's club.

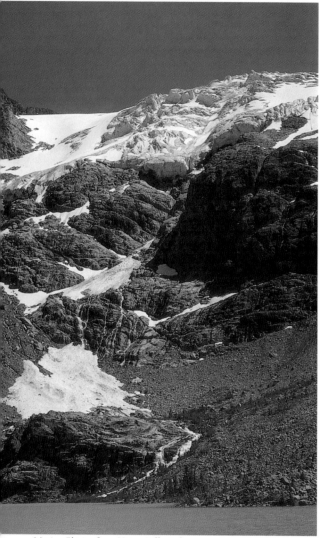

Matier Glacier from Upper Joffre Lake.

Continue your upward journey, and you'll emerge into bare talus slopes in full sun. Next is a bit more shade and overgrowth and another section of sweltering rockfall.

It might seem like forever, but it will actually only take 15 to 20 minutes before you espy Joffre Creek again. Not too much farther, the trail re-enters the cool respite of forest and shadows. A good spot for a break comes soon after, where a downed tree has been sliced into big chunks. Have a good long drink, rest your feet and soak your bandanna in the creek in preparation for the next upward section of trail.

At first steep, then gradual and rutted with exposed roots, this section can be a test of stamina, aerobic fitness and fancy footwork. But 30 slow steady minutes later, the trail levels out into subalpine forest. Through the trees is your first good glimpse of the Matier Glacier.

A few minutes of easy traversing and the trail drops to creek-side again. By way of a fallen-tree bridge, cross over and within moments Middle Joffre Lake is visible. At shore is a view that rivals any in the Rockies, with the lake's turquoise waters, virgin subalpine forest and the Matier Glacier spilling down in a frozen cascade between Joffre Peak and Slalok Mountain.

The trail skirts along the eastern shore of the lake then recrosses Joffre Creek. The first two bridges are nice big logs with hand railings, but take care on the second bridge—in summer the usual bridge is submerged so the crossing is made on a makeshift raft with no handholds. Once across, scramble under a fallen tree and up the talus slope in this poorly marked section, then into the trees.

As you ascend the last stretch of elevation, try to forget the upward grind and concentrate instead on the views of the creek, the lake and the distant peaks of the Cayoosh Range visible from the trail. Within 10 to 15 minutes, the trail levels out once again. A few minutes later, the trail brings you to the north end of Upper Joffre Lake, the largest, bluest and iciest of the three.

The trail winds along the western shore to the lake's south end where you'll likely see a few tents and bivouac bags pitched. Although it is possible to scramble among the talus slopes for closer views of the glacier, it's not recommended. Despite its solid presence, the glacier still releases tonnes of ice each summer. So, it's better to gaze on its icy grandeur from a respectful distance, out of the path of hurtling ice fall.

From there it's also easier to spot climbers navigating the icy perils above. Many of the features before you, as well as those hidden from view, were first climbed in the late 1950s by such mountaineering legends as Paddy Sherman. But some ascents went unchallenged until as recently as 1985.

Sit awhile and take in the sights. Once you're ready to tear yourself away from such sublime scenery, just retrace your steps to the parking area.

56 TENQUILLE LAKE

Distance: 12 km	Season: July to October
Elevation gain: 455 m	Topographical map:
High point: 1700 m	Birkenhead Lake 92J/10
Time needed: 5 hours	Trail map: Page 247
Rating: Moderate	

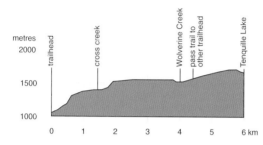

A T THE TURN OF THE 20TH CENTURY, prospectors saw the trails to Tenquille Lake as adits to hidden mineral riches. And although nobody got rich from the ventures, Tenquille Lake remains a treasure tucked high in the mountains above Pemberton. Old-growth forest, expansive alpine meadows and the turquoise beauty of the lake are the real riches to be discovered.

Two trails lead to Tenquille. One is a long, stiff hike from the Pemberton Valley; the other involves a bumpy drive along the Hurley River Forest Service Road and a rolling traverse. Our route takes the latter access.

To get to the trailhead, follow Highway 99 north to Pemberton. Zero the odometer at the T-junction and turn left towards the village of Pemberton, then follow the signs through town pointing to the Hurley River Road. A drive of almost 25 kilometres through the Pemberton Valley will bring you to the Hurley Road intersection. Turn right and follow the paved road to the bridge.

On the other side of the bridge the road turns to gravel, so if you have a 4x4, put it in gear at this point. (Also on the other side is the trailhead for the longer, stiffer hike to Tenquille.)

Just after the odometer clicks over to 33.5 kilometres, the road forks. Bear right onto the Hurley Road, towards Braelorne and Gold Bridge. Ten kilometres farther is a small wooden bridge and 700 metres past that a road branches to

Trail to Tenquille Lake, overlooking Pemberton Valley.

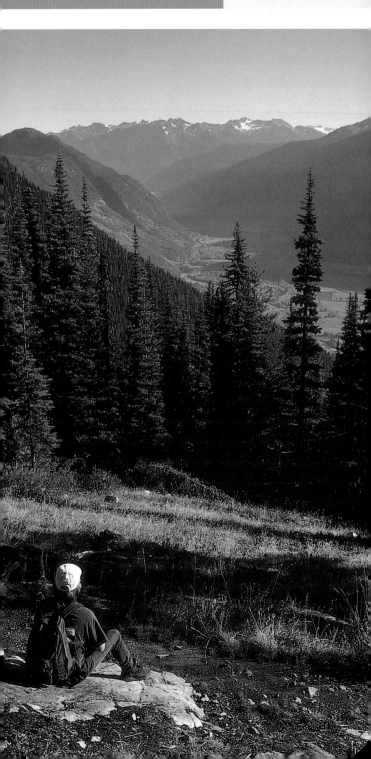

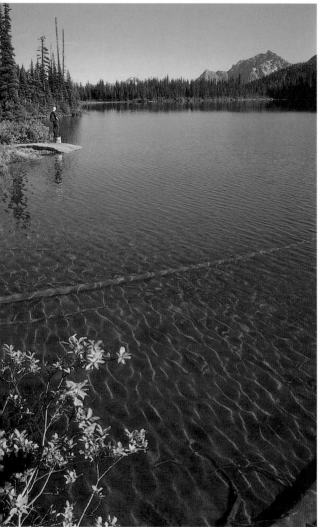

Tenquille Lake and Sun God Mountain.

the right. (There is a Tenquille Lake sign, somewhat obscured by brush.)

Recently, the Ministry of Forests pulled all the culverts out of this access road and installed water bars. Unless you have a four-wheel drive vehicle with moderate clearance, you'll need to park here and either bring a bike or hike the 5.5 kilometres to the trailhead proper. (And add another two hours to your hike time.) Whether you go on foot or on wheels, follow the road to a fork, then turn left. At the next fork (2.5 kilometres farther), go right. Another kilometre brings you to a parking area and the trailhead.

> The forest is so quiet that you can hear the bugs, the birds, the breeze, even your own heartbeat.

The end of the road features some spectacular views—a great way to start this scenic hike. The trail leads from the northeast corner of the parking area and climbs upwards, steeply at first, through an old clearcut now beginning to grow back.

Soon though, the trail enters a quiet forest of lichen-draped hemlock. And, a bit farther, where the trail passes through a saddle are black cottonwoods—unusual at this elevation, but perfectly at home in the moist conditions of this hollow. About 25 minutes from the start, the forest opens up, the trail takes a sharp switchback and rises to shadow the creek below.

Ignore the trail branching left a bit farther and continue on the main path as it drops from high above the north slopes of the creek to the creek itself. A stalwart bridge used to cross the creek—you can see parts of it washed out about 10 metres downstream—now, however, you must cross the creek by rock-hopping.

The trail rolls along through forest lined with mushrooms in autumn and with delicate woodland flowers in summer, through swamp and gully to emerge 20 minutes or so later to rock bluffs with great views across the valley.

Then it's down, down, down to another nameless creek, which you'll cross over a bridge. Ten minutes farther is another rustic bridge with a railing. Just beyond, the forest opens to reveal another viewpoint looking south to the farmlands of Pemberton Valley. Here, as well, there is a small creek to cross. Follow the pink tapes up a slighter higher trail that avoids the washout below.

The trail continues towards Wolverine Creek. Look up to see Goat Peak and, across the creek valley, the mountain called Copper Mound. The trail coming up from the Lillooet River is also visible on the distant meadowed slope. Ten minutes more brings the meeting of the trails. Continue straight up into expansive alpine meadows that, at the height of summer, are a sea of beautiful blue lupines and other wildflowers.

It's easy to spend hours exploring this vast boulder-strewn garden. If you do, keep to the trail and off the fragile vegetation. The thin soil and short-growing season in the alpine means such meadows can easily be damaged and take many, many years to recover, if at all.

The trail reaches the end of these alpine meadows about 35 to 40 minutes from the junction, then drops down through the pass. The lake soon becomes visible and within minutes, you're at the old cabin. The structure was built in the mid-1940s by a group of Pemberton residents, headed by Sandy Ross and Morgan Miller. Tenquille Lake was a favourite destination for families, but not many owned tents. So, the crew felled the amabilis fir nearby and packed in shingles on horseback for the roof. The windows, stove and many of the kitchen utensils, cutlery, tin plates and mugs were retrieved from abandoned mines in the area.

The names of visitors over the years have been etched into the cabin's timbers or recorded on pieces of metal. But a person has to wonder at the veracity of a record that reads 'Pierre Trudeau 80.'

The main trail leads farther to a Forest Service campsite for people staying overnight. Other trails wind to the lakeshore, the perfect place for a long lunch break and views of the surrounding mountains. Goat Peak lies to the northwest, the direction from which you came, and Tenquille Mountain is directly north.

Across the lake to the southwest is Copper Mound; directly south is Crown Mountain. In the distance to the southeast are Mounts Barbour and Ronayne and the ridges of Sun God Mountain.

The first miners seeking gold, silver and lead came to the Tenquille Lake area in 1909. By 1924, two trails had been established—one from the Pemberton Valley, called the John Jack Trail, and another from the railway, which today parallels the road to D'Arcy. (The latter trail isn't much used today as it is long and involves crossing several clearcuts.)

In the 1920s, the mountains surrounding Tenquille were riddled with mining claims that bore names such as Copper Dome, Silver Bell and Gold King. Near the summit of the 2130-metre Crown Mountain (then called McLeod), was a large cabin, two mine shafts and numerous trails leading to other sites. By 1929, most of the Tenquille Creek country had been staked.

These days, there is no mining activity. Just a lot of hikers, bikers and campers enjoying nature's treasures. After you've enjoyed, simply retrace your steps back to your vehicle.

PORT MOODY AREA

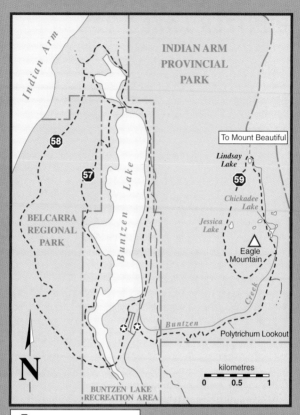

Indian Arm

INDIAN ARM
PROVINCIAL
PARK

To Mount Beautiful

*Lindsay
Lake*

59

*Chickadee
Lake*

*Jessica
Lake*

▲
Eagle
Mountain

Creek

58

57

Buntzen Lake

BELCARRA
REGIONAL
PARK

Buntzen

Polytrichum Lookout

N

kilometres
0   0.5   1

BUNTZEN LAKE
RECREATION AREA

---

57 Buntzen Lake, p. 262
58 Sendero Diez Vistas, p. 266
59 Eagle Ridge, p. 270

57 BUNTZEN LAKE

Distance: 10 km	Rating: Easy
Elevation gain: Minimal	Season: Year-round
High point: 250 m	Topographical map:
Time needed: 4 hours	Port Coquitlam 92G/7
	Trail map: Page 261

Note: Dogs must be leashed. In wet weather, bring an extra pair of shoes.

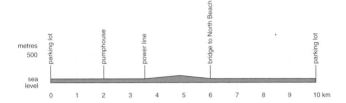

D URING SUMMER, THE SHORES OF Buntzen Lake swell with Coquitlamites looking for a cool place to beat the heat. For the other three seasons of the year though, the trails surrounding Buntzen Lake are a perfect hiking getaway—close enough to the city for easy access, but far enough away and filled with the soothing sights of lake, marsh, forest and mountain.

To get to the starting point, first head to Port Moody. Turn north from the Lougheed Highway onto Ioco Road and follow the signs pointing to Buntzen Lake. Bear right at Parkside Drive and into the Heritage Mountain subdivision. At East Road, turn left. At Sunnyside Road, turn right and continue to the main parking lot at Buntzen.

The trailhead proper is at the southwest corner of the lot. The trail meanders through a short section of forest, then crosses the marshy end of the lake on a wooden footbridge. Once over the bridge, turn right onto the gravel road and watch for horses. In some places—such as this—hikers share the trail with horseback riders as well as mountain bikers, so be prepared for galloping hoofs and the occasional pile of horse droppings.

The gravel trail ends at a pumphouse intake. Look to the left for the Buntzen Lake Trail—for hikers only—which leads into the woods. The trail wanders lakeside for the first while, then heads upwards into a forest of cedar, hemlock and fir. (In wetter weather, the trail can get pretty muddy, so bring a clean, dry pair of après-hike shoes.)

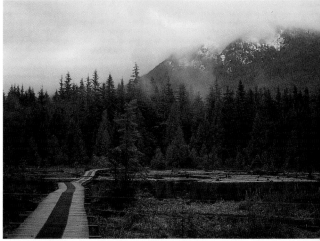

Floating walkway across south end of Buntzen Lake.

Some sections are steepish, but there's nothing too strenuous or long-lasting. Soon the sounds of a nearby stream trickle in and, not much further, the path splits. Stay to the left.

The trail eventually wanders onto open bluffs directly under the power line. From here, there is a great view of the lake and of Eagle Ridge looming opposite. Not visible is the 5-metre-wide, 4-kilometre-long tunnel that brings water from Coquitlam Lake to Buntzen Lake. The tunnel was blasted through the solid granite of Eagle Ridge in 1903 as part of the Vancouver Power Company's first hydroelectric project to provide electricity to Vancouver. Previously, the city's power supply came from a steam plant.

The system is still in use. Water pours from Coquitlam Lake via the underground aqueduct into the north end of Buntzen Lake. Water from Buntzen then flows through penstocks down the precipitous slopes of Indian Arm to the two powerhouses below. The first powerhouse was built in 1903 and modernized in 1951; the second was built in 1914. Together, they still put out 145 megawatts annually—enough to supply power to 14,500 homes each year.

Reel in that knowledge and plop down for a lunch break—best if the sun is shining. Once ready to push on, pick your way down among a jumble of loose rock to the north end of the lake, being careful to watch your footing. From the small cable suspension bridge, look north to see another pumphouse intake. Cross the bridge to reach the grass, picnic tables and outhouses at the lake's North Beach.

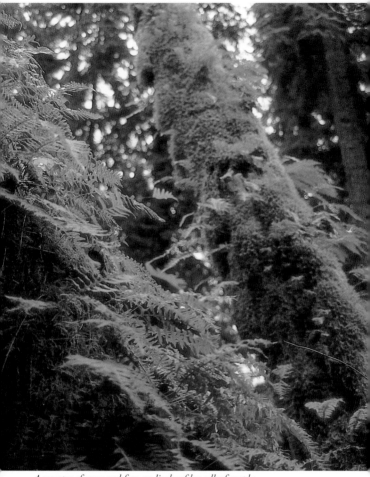

A sweater of moss and fern on limbs of broadleaf maple.

Before it was called Buntzen Lake—after Johannes Buntzen, the first general manager of the BC Electric Railway Company—the water before you was called 'Lake Beautiful' by the Native Peoples who lived in the area.

The lake figures prominently in coastal lore. There once was a time, according to Coast Salish legend, when it rained and rained and rained. After many weeks of constant rainfall, the levels of the streams, rivers, lakes and seas began to rise. The people gathered at the only place considered safe from the advancing waters—the shoreline of Lake Beautiful.

A council was held and a decision made that a great canoe be built and a long cedar lash woven to anchor the craft if the water continued to rise. All the people laboured without sleep to complete the task. And then, as Pauline Johnson recounts in her 1911 book *Legends of Vancouver*:

> Noble hands lifted every child of the tribe into this vast canoe; not one single baby was overlooked. The canoe was stocked with food and fresh water, and lastly, the ancient men and women of the race selected as guardians to these children the bravest, most stalwart, handsomest young man of the tribe, and the mother of the youngest baby in camp
> —she was but a girl of 16, but she, too, was brave and very beautiful.

The two took their posts in the craft, the young man at the stern to guide, the young woman at the bow to watch; the children crowded between the two.

> And still the sea crept up, and up, and up. At the crest of the bluffs about Lake Beautiful, the doomed tribes crowded. Not a single person attempted to enter the canoe. There was no wailing, no crying out.

The waters folded over the bluffs, the people and the top of the tallest tree, then all was water. After days and days afloat, held fast by a cedar lash to an enormous boulder underwater, the pair espied distant land—the summit of Mount Baker. They cut the lash, drifted south and landed on Baker's slopes, now bared by the receding waters. And life went on.

It's something to ponder on the walk back along the eastern shoreline trail, where brooks burble through moss-covered rocks, past aspens and birches and into the sparkling lake. Canoeists and kayakers dip their paddles in the tranquillity of the season. The occasional fisherman casts a line in search of cutthroat trout, Dolly Varden char, kokanee and other species with which the lake is stocked.

Eventually, the trail emerges from the woods to South Beach and the parking lot where you started.

58 SENDERO DIEZ VISTAS

Distance: 15 km	Rating: Moderate
Elevation gain: 440 m	Season: April to November
High point: 560 m	Topographical map:
Time needed: 6–7 hours	Port Coquitlam 92G/7
	Trail map: Page 261

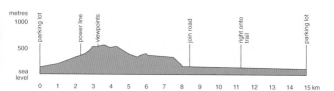

ONE OF THE PRETTIEST TRAILS IN THE Lower Mainland exists only because of the efforts of master trail builder Halvor Lunden. Named Sendero Diez Vistas (in Spanish, Ten Viewpoints Trail), after its splendid lookouts of Indian Arm and the Fannin Range, it has been a well-kept secret among Lower Mainland hikers for years.

Halvor first began work on the trail about 15 years ago, surveying, clearing brush by hand and marking the route. The only thing he didn't have to clear were the viewpoints. 'When I build a trail, I try to disturb an area as little as possible,' says Halvor. 'It's much nicer the way nature makes it.'

Start the hike from the north end of the main parking lot at Buntzen Lake, following a signed trail into the woods and across a wooden footbridge over a marshy end of the lake. On the other side, the trail meets with a service road. Cross it and follow the signs dead ahead pointing the way to Diez Vistas trail.

For the next 40 minutes or so, the path leads upwards at a steady respectable pace through second-growth forest. Then comes a fork in the trail. Stay left and continue heading up. A few minutes later, the trail splits in three directions. Go straight, towards the power lines and under the pipeline. (The pipeline, no longer in use, once fed water from the Buntzen reservoir to the Burrard Thermal Plant below.)

As the trail zigs and zags its way up to Buntzen Ridge, it allows occasional glimpses of Burrard Inlet to the west. Here's a geological fun fact: Had the Capilano Dam not been built, trapping sediments from the Capilano River, the passage under Lions Gate Bridge would have narrowed, and Burrard Inlet would eventually have become Burrard Lake.)

Near the top of the ridge, the trail bears sharply right to the

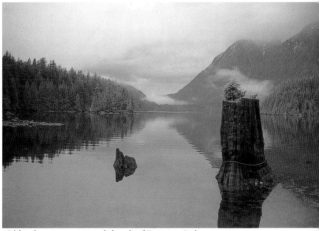

Old cedar snag near south beach of Buntzen Lake.

first really great viewpoint (although not one of the official 10). From the aptly named Punta Largueza, or Appreciation Point, hikers can see power boats and sailboats scoot like waterbugs into Belcarra Bay, and watch rafts of kayakers learning the basics near the shores of Jug and Raccoon islands. And you may be able to pick out picnickers on the shores of Sasamat Lake. After the upward grind, this viewpoint is also a good place to take a well-deserved water break.

From here, the trail winds north. In another few minutes, there's another view, this time of Buntzen Lake and the forests you climbed through. Another few minutes, and it's Punta del Este, with its views east of Buntzen's south beach, and of Eagle Ridge, with the recently named Halvor Lunden Trail.

About 10 minutes farther, the trail veers left, then heads up. You'll know you're on the right track when you spot the sign noting the Valley Outdoor Association's adoption of the trail and a little farther, the sign for Sendero Diez Vistas. Follow the path as it drops down from the high part of the ridge to a swampy saddle, then rises to the ridge's north side for Viewpoint #1.

From here, and the next nine lookouts, your views are of the Fannin Range, much of it contained within Mount Seymour Provincial Park. In late spring and early summer, snow may still cover the cols and peaks of Mounts Seymour, Elsay and Bishop. And snowmelt may been seen cascading down the steep slopes along Scott-Goldie, Percy and Shone creeks.

Much of those lower slopes are now included in Indian Arm Provincial Park. Created in 1995, the park also includes

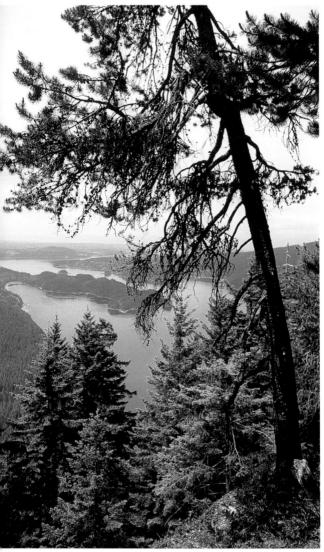

From the first viewpoint – Punta Largueza.

significant amounts of land on the eastern side of Indian Arm. A planning process is currently underway to map out the park's future. One of the ideas being talked about is a trail that would wrap entirely around Indian Arm, from North Vancouver to Belcarra.

Muse a little on this dream trail before continuing on to Viewpoints #2 through #10, taking in the sunny vistas and the cool shadows of the forest. After Viewpoint #10, the trail begins its lakeward descent. Along the way are remnants of logging history—a cable anchor, skid roads and big stumps. Where the trail emerges into a sylvan glade, go left. About 15 minutes after having left the ridge top, you'll emerge onto a service road with absolutely no signs anywhere.

> Although trees here were harvested early in the 20th century, a few big Douglas firs remain. Their lower trunks have been scarred black by a long-ago fire, but they still stand straight and tall.

If you feel like heading back, go right to a water intake, then right again to follow the trail over the wooden suspension bridge to Buntzen's North Beach. It's an hour's easy walking from here along the east lakeshore trail to the parking lot.

But, for an additional 30-minute side-trip of some big old trees, penstocks and an island-dotted lake, go left to follow the Lakeview Trail. Blowdown has blocked the trail in places, so go here only if your route-finding skills are solid. A few minutes later should bring you to a paved road on which you'll head right towards the big penstocks that carry water from Buntzen to the powerhouses on Indian Arm below.

As the road swings south, you'll walk along the shore of a smaller lake. On some maps, it's called Trout Lake—actually one of Buntzen Lake's earlier names. But others believe it would be more appropriate to call the water body McCombe Lake after the McCombe family—Bob, Sarah, Mona and Bob Jr.—who lived beside the lake from 1911 to 1929. Bob McCombe was the foreman of the Tunnel Camp, which blasted a 4-kilometre-long tunnel from Coquitlam Lake to Buntzen Lake via the solid granite of Eagle Ridge. The island in the lake's centre is known as Mona Island after perhaps its most ardent admirer—Mona McCombe.

Eventually, the lake fades from view and the road leads to the North Beach picnic area on Buntzen and an easy hour's walking along the east lakeshore trail to the south beach and the parking lot.

59 EAGLE RIDGE

Distance: 15 km	Season: Late June to October
Elevation gain: 1020 m	Topographical map:
High point: 1130 m	Port Coquitlam 92G/7
Time needed: 6.5–7 hours	Trail map: Page 261
Rating: Strenuous	

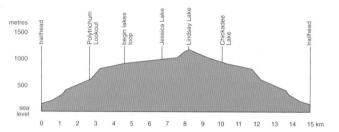

SUBURBAN GROWTH MAY BE CREEPING farther up the mountainside in Port Moody, edging ever closer to Buntzen Lake, but there are still wild places in the area to retreat to when you need to get away from it all but can't get out of the Lower Mainland.

From the lakeshore, Eagle Ridge is striking enough as the wall of granite and trees that forms the dramatic eastern backdrop to Buntzen Lake. But way up high, the ridge holds other treasures—magnificent views of the Lower Mainland, tiny jewel-like lakes and an outstanding grove of old-growth forest.

A word of warning though: The hike is not for beginners or for the less than fit. It's a stiff trip where every footstep forward seems to take you another metre higher. Although it is theoretically possible to do a 10-hour, 25-kilometre loop of the entire ridge, we'll restrict ourselves to a scenic 15-kilometre loop.

Virtually all the trails in the Buntzen area have been built by Halvor Lunden. Now in his 80s, Halvor still comes out on the weekends

> Giant yellow cedars predominate. Although many have been topped by the elements, their girths are similar to that of the Point Atkinson Lighthouse. I measured one yellow cedar on the trail at more than 7 metres in circumference.

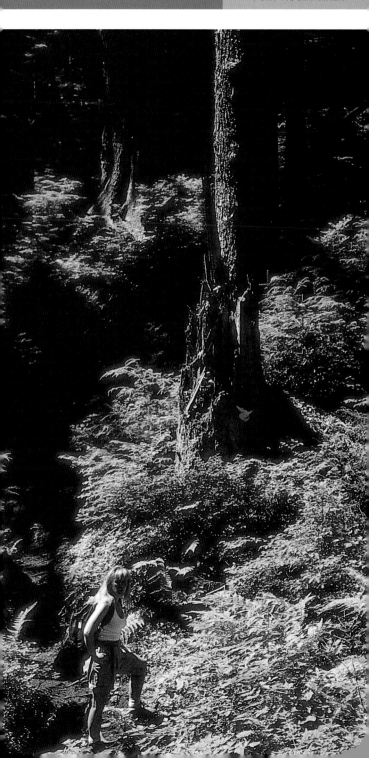

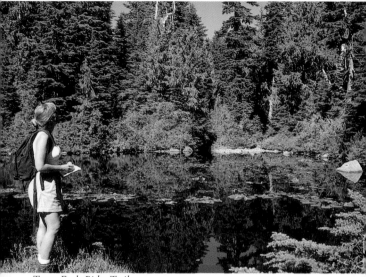

Tarns, Eagle Ridge Trail.

to maintain them, toting a heavy pack of tools and bounding up the trail faster than most 20-year-olds. In 1996, Halvor's long-time efforts were rewarded by BC Hydro and BC Parks, and he had a trail officially named after him. It is here that today's hike starts.

The trailhead is on the Powerhouse Road, just east of the southeasternmost corner of the main parking lot. (Look for the yellow gate.) At the trailhead is a sign noting Halvor's trail-building contributions and a map showing the paths he's hewn over the years.

Go straight ahead to take the Halvor Lunden Trail, which winds through second-growth forest. In autumn, the slender vine maples here burst into a blaze of colour against the moss-draped background of larger broadleaf maples and giant ferns. The occasional big stump hints at the size of the original conifers.

Within a few minutes, the path crosses a wooden bridge over a seasonal creek and begins its ascent. In another few minutes, the trail comes to a T-junction. Go left into the open area under the power lines.

A few minutes of hiking past fireweed and other flora common to disturbed areas brings you to a wooden signpost. Bear right and follow the familiar orange diamonds and tape into the cool of the forest.

The trail climbs steadily and relentlessly for 35 to 40 minutes before levelling out for a 5- to 10-minute gentler walk through a grove of larger trees, still second-growth, punctuated by the burned snags and stumps of the original forest. Then it's back to the steady and relentless uphill hike.

Finally, 20 minutes or so later, is Polytrichum Lookout, named after *Polytrichum juniperinum,* a verdant moss that grows in the vicinity. From here, Mount Elsay and the three peaks of Mount Seymour form a backdrop to views of Vancouver and Burnaby in the hazy distance, Buntzen Ridge directly across and Buntzen Lake below.

Both the lake and one of the summits on Eagle Ridge used to go by the name of Beautiful. The lake was renamed in honour of Johannes Buntzen, the first general manager of the BC Electric Railway Company. The summit was dubbed Eagle Peak but that name was too close to the name of another summit—Eagle Mountain. Efforts are underway to restore the original Beautiful name.

After a good rest, continue the ascent through the forest, eventually emerging into a ravine through which Buntzen Creek flows. Here, the trail leads through a stately grove of old-growth trees—western red cedar, spruce, Douglas fir, yellow cedar.

Then, for contrast, the trail tops out and emerges into an area that looks at first like a big clearcut but is actually several swathes cut between 15 and 20 years ago. Fireweed and blueberry bush now proliferate, making it good bear habitat. Be sure to make lots of noise when trundling along.

The trail follows the perimeter of the clearcut for 20 minutes or so, right to a cliff's edge. Only a tree's width remains between the cliff edge and the cut. Eventually, the trail leads back into the trees and a few minutes farther arrives at El Paso Junction. At this point, you are actually standing on an old dyke. What appears to be a steep-walled creek before you was once an aqueduct built in the 1920s to supply water from Noons Creek to Port Moody.

Go left to follow the way signposted 'Lindsay Lake via viewpoints,' across the creek/aqueduct, and clamber up the opposite bank into one of the most beautiful old-growth forests in the Lower Mainland.

Thirty minutes of walking through this verdant treasure brings you to the first of the viewpoints—Barton Point. From here is a view of virtually the entire Lower Mainland. On many hot, sunny days, though, you won't be able to see the city for the haze. With luck, Mount Baker and Mount Shuksan will gleam high and white above the thick brown urban blanket.

After almost three hours on the trail, you'll be tempted to stop here for lunch. But I suggest pushing on another 15 minutes to Little Valhalla viewpoint, where the view is nicer and the setting more secluded.

Five to 10 minutes past Little Valhalla is a trail junction. If you're uncomfortable with heights, go right and take the bypass. But for a short diversion well worth the time and effort, go left to the viewpoint at Spahats Rigg or Bear Ridge—so named by Halvor because of the preponderance of bears there when he first worked the trail. A 10-minute scramble up a steepish rock bluff affords views of distant peaks, such as Coliseum and the Camel, which can't be seen from the lower lookouts.

Continue over the bump and drop back down into the trees to meet the main trail again. Just a bit farther is Jessica Lake, actually more of a lily pond, named by Halvor after the tiny Texas tot who tumbled into a well and captured world attention in 1987.

Ten minutes farther, the trail takes an abrupt right—just before a big rock outcrop—and climbs. A few minutes later is the West Point lookout and just beyond that, a flat rock outcrop called The Pulpit. The trail veers away from the ridge's west side and heads uphill, emerging to peeks of Lindsay Lake and a major trail junction. To the left the trail continues uphill for another 2.8 kilometres to Mount Beautiful (aka Eagle Peak) and beyond to Swan Falls and Dilly Dally Peak.

We, however, follow the loop trail along the lakeshore and into the subalpine meadows. The path descends through thickets of berry bushes, stunted trees and pondlets, eventually running alongside Nancy Catch Creek.

Within 10 to 15 minutes, you'll reach a junction. The trails to the east and west lead to longer, less well-marked routes that pass unremarkable lakelets. So it's best to stay straight ahead on the main trail, which takes you past the yellow water-lily blooms of Chickadee Lake, then past the smaller but sweetly scenic Siskin and Wren Lakes.

Eventually, the trails all merge and lead down, down, down, past Foy Falls to the El Paso Junction where your ridge walk began. Just head straight out and retrace the rest of your steps along the cliff edge, through the clearcut, past Polytrichum Lookout, and down, down, down to the parking lot.

PORT COQUITLAM AREA

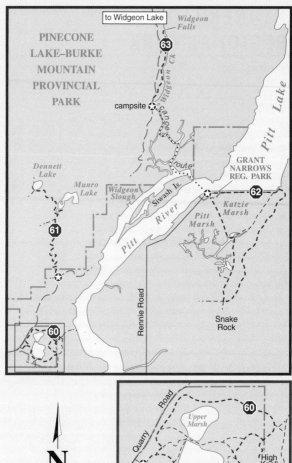

to Widgeon Lake

Widgeon Falls

63

PINECONE
LAKE–BURKE
MOUNTAIN
PROVINCIAL
PARK

Widgeon Ck

campsite

canoe

route

GRANT
NARROWS
REG. PARK

62

Dennett
Lake

Munro
Lake

Widgeon
Slough

Siwash Is.

Pitt River

Katzie
Marsh

61

Pitt
Marsh

Pitt Lake

Rennie Road

Snake
Rock

60

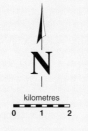

N

kilometres

0   1   2

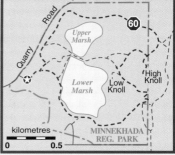

Quarry Road

Upper
Marsh

60

Lower
Marsh

Low
Knoll

High
Knoll

MINNEKHADA
REG. PARK

kilometres

0   0.5

60 Minnekhada, p. 276
61 Munro and Dennett Lakes, p. 280
62 Pitt Wildlife Loop, p. 284
63 Widgeon Falls, p. 288

60 MINNEKHADA REGIONAL PARK

Distance: 11 km	Rating: Easy
Elevation gain: Minimal	Season: Year-round
High point: 150 m	Topographical map:
Time needed: 3 hours	Coquitlam 92G/7
	Trail map: Page 275

Note: Dogs must be leashed. Bring binoculars for birdwatching.

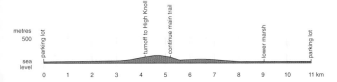

WHEN HIGHER MOUNTAIN ROUTES ARE still hidden by snow and ice, there are still some lower elevation destinations that are perfect as a hiking warm-up or for introducing new hikers to the great outdoors.

Minnekhada Regional Park is such a place. Within the 175-hectare park are 10 kilometres of trails; just adjoining are another 15 or so kilometres of trail that circle the Pitt-Addington Marsh Wildlife Management Area.

The terrain is varied—from long, flat stretches of dyke to rollicking forest trail to the High Knoll, with its fabulous views of the Fraser Valley. There's enough tramping to keep a stalwart hiker happy. And, at the same time, there are shorter loop trails perfect for beginning hikers, families and kids.

Our route starts at Quarry Road parking lot on the park's north side. The shortest loop covers about 11 kilometres and takes about two to three hours. The longest version covers more than 25 kilometres in total and will take six to eight hours.

To get to the starting point, follow the Lougheed Highway to Port Coquitlam. Turn north on Coast Meridian Road and follow the green and yellow park signs. (Turn right on Apel Drive, and right again on Victoria Drive until it forks left and becomes the gravel of Quarry Road.) The park entrance is on the right, roughly 3.5 kilometres from the fork.

After parking in the Quarry Road lot, tramp along the Lodge Trail for about 100 metres then bear left to the Meadow Trail, which you'll follow to the next fork. Take Quarry Trail. From

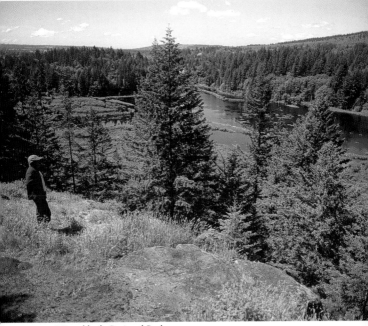

Minnekhada Regional Park.

here, we'll walk under the arms of fragrant red alder along the park's northwestern perimeter.

If tree limbs are bare, you'll see Quarry Road. There is a good viewpoint of the Upper Marsh, and just a bit farther, the North Trail, which winds along the park's northern boundary.

Minnekhada Regional Park is part of what was once a 670-hectare farm owned by wealthy Vancouver lumber entrepreneur Harry Jenkins in the 1900s. It is believed that Jenkins brought the name with him when he left Minneapolis, Minnesota in 1904. Derived from the Sioux language, Minnekhada means 'beside running waters.' In 1918, Jenkins left the farm because of economic and health woes. Eventually, the land was bought by lumber magnate and soon-to-be lieutenant-governor Eric Hamber. More about him later.

Eventually, the trail levels off. A breeze often rustles the boughs of cedar above, giving more reason to contemplate this regional gem, only a short walk and drive from suburbia.

The trail descends gradually to the bottom of a hill where you're faced with a decision. Do you bear left for a 15-kilometre, three- to four-hour-long journey on the Addington Loop Trail as it winds around the dyked perimeter of the Pitt–Addington

> The way gradually rises into a mixed forest of alder and maple, cedar and fir. Water trickles down rocky outcrops, making perfect little rock gardens of moss, flower and fern.

Marsh? Or do you head right towards High Knoll and the marshes of the park?

(If you do go left, there is also the option of a slightly higher route that wanders for about 30 minutes along a ridge, with views of the marsh and points beyond, before looping back to the Panabode Trail.)

However, since I'm always such a sucker for the big views, we'll bear right and follow the trail to the modest heights of High Knoll—a 150-metre-high rocky prominence. It's the perfect place for a lunch with a view: Pitt River and the farmlands of Pitt Meadows to the east, Golden Ears and other Coastal Range peaks farther on and, if you're lucky enough to have a haze-free day, even the dormant volcano of Mount Baker.

Once you've had enough, descend to the junction and head left on the Triangle Trail. About 200 metres farther, the trail forks. Go right if you've had enough for the day. A 40-minute walk will take you across the dyke dividing the upper and lower marshes, along the Meadows Trail to the parking lot.

Even if you're keen for more, it's worth taking a look at the marsh before moving on. Before the Pitt River was dyked in the 1890s, Minnekhada lay in the river floodplain. Each spring, snowmelt swelled the river, leaving the area temporarily underwater. Things dried out after the dykes were built. Later work in the 1930s and '40s divided the area into an upper and lower marsh. Then beavers moved in and decided to do a little dyking of their own. From time to time, Ducks Unlimited comes in to deconstruct some of the beaver dams and keep the marsh habitable for all the bird species found there.

Once you've taken that in, return to the fork you came by and head left and, a bit farther, left again. Just a bit farther beyond is a T-junction. The right trail leads to Low Knoll. But when you've already been high, the temptation will be to go left and follow the contours of the forest to an intersection with the Panabode Trail.

Pass up the opportunity to head for Addington Marsh and go right here to follow a section of trail that seems charmed— with the twittering of songbirds, the subtle views of the lower marsh and an air of tranquillity.

Eventually, you'll come to a picnic area, just north of the Minnekhada Lodge, which was built in 1934 as a country retreat and hunting lodge by lumber baron and Lieutenant-Governor Eric Hamber.

Polo matches were once popular here, as were duck and pheasant hunting. And famous folk such as Princess Elizabeth of England and Prince Bernhardt of The Netherlands stayed as guests at the lodge. The Hambers apparently also kept a resident and official welcoming monkey who delighted guests by pinching bananas from a fruit bowl.

If you want to look inside, come when the Greater Vancouver Regional District holds an open house. There's always one on the first Sunday of each month between 1 and 4 PM. On other Sundays, there may be an open house, but it depends on bookings. For more information, phone CVRD Parks at (604) 432-6350.

From here, it's just a short walk along the edges of the lower marsh—bring binoculars to get a good look at all the birds—and onto the Lodge Trail back to the parking lot.

61 MUNRO & DENNETT LAKES

Distance: 11 km	Rating: Moderate
Elevation gain: 880 m	Season: June to October
High point: 955 m	Topographical map:
Time needed: 6 hours	Port Coquitlam 92G/7
	Trail map: Page 275

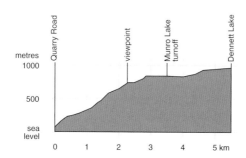

O LD-GROWTH TREES, VIEWPOINTS, interesting marshy bits and two pretty little lakes await you on the trail to Munro and Dennett Lakes. Hiking this trail used to involve technical trespass on private property (although none of the hundreds of hikers who did so was ever charged).

Now, however, that circumstance is all part of the past. In 1995, the provincial government declared the area a 'Class A' park: the Pinecone Lake/Burke Mountain Provincial Park as it is formally and cumbersomely known.

The study team that set aside the provincial park where this hike takes us considered Burke Mountain a rare feature in the Lower Mainland, because of its subalpine meadows, numerous ponds and lakes, and long, gentle ridge.

So get out there and hit the legal trail. But first, to the trailhead. Take the Lougheed Highway to Port Coquitlam and turn left on Coast Meridian Road, following the signs towards Minnekhada Regional Park. At Apel Road turn right and, at Victoria Drive, turn right again. Where the road splits, stay on the left fork until you hit the gravel of Quarry Road.

Soon, you'll see the signs to Minnekhada, but don't turn, just keep following the road straight ahead. About 3.5 kilometres farther, look on the left for the Burke Mountain sign, tucked into the bushes. This point is the start. Park off the side of the road in the well-used pullouts.

Wetlands near Dennett Lake.

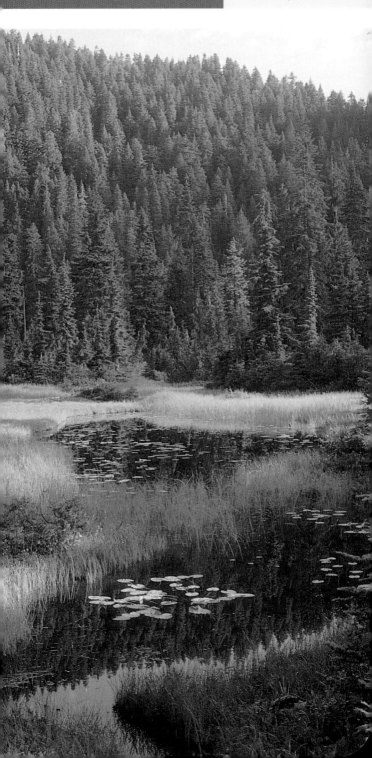

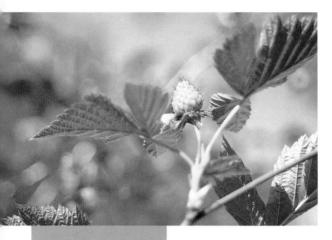

If you head up the trail in early summer, you'll be greeted by thickets of salmonberry bushes with ripe yellow and red berries just begging you to pick and eat them.

Look for some orangey-red ties on the right that mark your route. Carved faintly into an accompanying tree is the word MUNRO and an arrow pointing right. Follow it.

Head uphill, following the orange and red diamond-shaped trail markers. A mere 10 minutes later, the trail splits. If you go to the left, you'll find a tumble of mini-waterfalls and swimming pools. Be careful, the rocks are very, very slippery. But do take 15 minutes to explore and poke around.

Then, rejoin the trail again and follow it up. Every once in a while, the trail splits, then a little further up, rejoins. For the sake of continuity, stay left. About an hour after your start, a short side-trail leads to the right and views of the Pitt River and surrounding farmlands. Another 15 minutes brings another viewpoint, this time with a glimpse of the working quarry on the west side of the river. Where the trail passes a small rock slide, another vantage pops into view, this one looking down to Minnekhada Park and its easily recognized High Knoll.

Then it's back to the steady slog uphill. Most of the trees you'll pass are second-growth. Portions of Burke Mountain were logged early in the 20th century. During the 1920s and '30s, fire damaged other stands. Still, the mountain has one of the most southerly unfragmented mature forests in the Lower Mainland.

A little higher, the trail levels to an area characterized more by mud, swamp and skunk cabbage than by awe-inspiring trees. Look for the sign, nailed way up high on a tree, which points the way to Munro Lake. Follow the pink ties as you scramble over exposed roots and rocks. Soon you'll come to the lakeshore.

Munro Lake was once dammed to provide water for an old quarry near the Pitt River. The dam has now been removed and the lake has returned to its natural level. Before the dam was breached, the lake was stocked with eastern brook trout, which made it a popular fishing spot.

For years, the area was owned by Genstar Development Company. At one point, a hotel/condominium development with downhill ski facilities was proposed for the area. (Locals familiar with the here-today, gone-tomorrow nature of snow on Burke must have laughed themselves silly.)

The lake is much larger than it looks at first glimpse. Head right along the shore to get a better look. There are many spots worth stopping for a break before you continue to Dennett Lake.

After a rest, return to the point where you first approached the lakeshore and follow the lake's west side. Watch for tiny little frogs; they're everywhere among the mud and marsh. Cross over a couple of feeder streams, then after a few minutes, just past a twisted tree standing all alone, you'll come to a real creek.

Head into the forest at the tapes, go past the campfire remnants, cross the creek and follow the tapes. The trail soon heads upward and steepens for about 15 minutes of hiking. The rest of the way involves more wading than hiking, through swampy meadows and creeks. Soon, a teeny tiny, nameless lake passes your vision—but this is not Dennett. Just keep going, following the ties, and soon, you'll see it—a beautiful blue jewel of a lake, set against a backdrop of sheer cliffs.

This scenery is some of what sets Burke apart as a mountain. According to BC Parks, there are few other places within the Southern Pacific Ranges Ecosection with such broad subalpine plateaus. That's part of the reason the province created the park. Trail maintenance, signage and better facilities will likely come as a result of the park's Class A status, but it will probably take a while. So, enjoy the views, have a dip in the chilly waters and rest easy knowing that this special place is now protected.

When you're done, retrace your steps back to Quarry Road.

62 PITT WILDLIFE LOOP

Distance: 12 km	Rating: Moderate
Elevation gain: 150 m	Season: Year-round
High point: 150 m	Topographical map:
Time needed: Up to 5 hours	Port Coquitlam 92G/7
	Trail map: Page 275

Note: Bring binoculars for birdwatching.

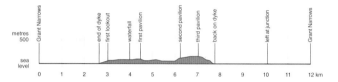

S OME OF THE BEST HIKES ARE THE ONES FEW
people know about. For example, most people know
the Pitt Polder area for the kilometres of flat, wide
dykes, which are great walking and birdwatching venues. But
few people ever wander the slopes east of the marsh along the
Mountainside Trail, with its waterfalls, sumptuous forest and
stunning views.

A word of warning: Technically (i.e., for liability reasons) the
mountainside trails are considered "closed." In reality, they're
quite manageable, although sometimes not in the best condition.
Some bridges are broken, some sections are overgrown, others
are rough and/or slippery. If you find the trails unsuitable for
your abilities, a long walk on the marsh dykes can provide you
with a long, long walk with lots to see.

Our route, which makes for about five hours of moderate,
leisurely hiking, begins at Grant Narrows. To get there, follow
the Lougheed Highway to Pitt Meadows. Just after you've
crossed the Pitt River Bridge, turn left onto Dewdney Trunk
Road, then left again on Harris Road, right on McNeil and
left on Rannie Road, which you will follow to its end—the
aforementioned narrows.

Park in the lot, then head east along dyke that marks the
southern boundary of Pitt Lake, the largest freshwater tidal lake
in North America. Because it's so close to the point where the
Fraser River meets the Pacific Ocean, water levels rise and fall
with the tides. Thousands of years ago Pitt Lake was a saltwater
fjord, much like nearby Indian Arm, but as the Fraser River
deposited more and more sediment, the Pitt waters were cut
off from the sea.

After 25 to 30 minutes of walking, the dyke ends. Continue

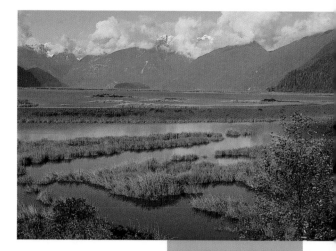

past where Swan Dyke turns south, past the old sections of wooden board lying in the grass. The access to the mountainside trail isn't obvious. The wooden bridge that once carried hikers to the trailhead has been removed. It is still possible to hop down and walk the 5 metres or so to the trailhead, but it can be rather wet at times.

On sunny days, Pitt Lake is resplendent; on cloudy days, it's cloaked in mystery with wispy tendrils of mist wrapping around the trees, islands and cliffs.

Just look for the square silver marker nailed to a tree; it and its look-alikes will be your guides throughout the hike.

Only 10 to 15 minutes from the trailhead is the first lookout—worth a scoot for a quick look, but the views are better farther along.

The trail meanders through the trees and creekbeds and, 20 to 30 minutes later, comes to a waterfall. A short side-trail leads to a view of a white veil of water tumbling over tiers of mossy, lichen-covered rock. It's as good a reason as you'll ever need for a water break.

After the falls, backtrack to the last marker (on a tree near the fallen tree just before you cross a small creek). Then scramble up a short rocky section and continue moseying. Within 30 minutes, the trail arrives at the first of three wooden pavilions on the trail. From here, all of Katzie Marsh lies before you. The Pitt River snakes its way west to Widgeon Slough and south to the Fraser River.

Then, the trail heads down, down, down the slope to marsh

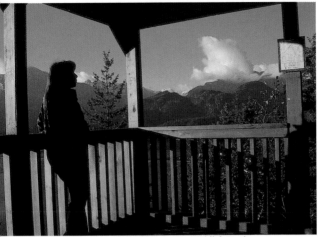

Distant peaks, from the lookout on Pitt Wildlife Trail.

level, among moss-covered trees. Some of the cedar stumps along the way are sizeable—4 to 5 metres around. Close your eyes and try to imagine how tall they once must have stood.

Twenty minutes of hiking brings you to a fork in the trail. Uphill leads to another waterfall, well worth the short side-trip. Straight ahead leads to an open area where it's possible to call it a day, cross the bridge to Swan Dyke and head for the narrows.

We, however, will push on for another 40 to 50 minutes of moderate elevation gain to the second pavilion, perched about 100 metres above sea level on a rock bluff. From this vantage is a stunning 180° view of the entire area—farmlands and Sheridan Hill to the south, Burke Ridge and Coquitlam Mountain to the west, Pitt Lake to the North.

Way before the arrival of non-Natives, this area was home to the Katzie people. It still is—one of four present-day reserves is directly across Grant Narrows. The Katzie ancestors harvested area plants for food and medicine, hunted waterfowl in the marshes and had special spiritual places on the shores of Pitt Lake.

But long, long ago, according to Katzie mythology, there were no animals yet in the world. Swaneset, the Supreme Benefactor, was first sent by the Creator Spirit. He created the first sturgeon and a white owl. He introduced seagulls and eulachon and brought sockeye salmon from far away.

Then, notes Katzie chief Old Pierre in the 1955 book *The Faith of a Coast Salish Indian,* came Khaals, one of 3 brothers sent to finish Swaneset's work. As the brothers travelled from the west along the Lower Fraser Valley, they transformed people into wolves, mink, kingfishers and other animals. When they reached Sheridan Hill, Khaals changed one man into a steelhead salmon, others to Salish suckers, beavers, muskrats and geese. Next, he came upon two sisters digging up potatoes from the mud. 'Do you eat these potatoes?' he asked. 'Yes,' they replied, 'we have nothing else to eat.'

'Very well,' he said, 'you shall become sandhill cranes. Henceforth you shall roam over the meadows as you do now.' He raised his hand and transformed the sisters. So now cranes laugh and dance after they root up the ground, just as the two sisters laughed and danced as they dug up their potatoes.

At certain times of year, sandhill cranes still return to the marsh to dig in the ground, laugh and dance. If you're lucky you'll see one. Otherwise, take in the views, have lunch, then regain the main trail as it heads downslope. After 45 minutes or so, the trail meets a side-trail to the third pavilion.

If you've only got enough energy to complete the 30 to 40 minutes of dyke walking back to the car, you may want to pass. Otherwise, slog up the steep trail for 15 minutes or so to the third pavilion, well worth the effort. As the southernmost pavilion, it has the best views south, of Burnt Hill, the Pitt River and surrounding farmlands. It's also perched the highest, at 150 metres.

Finally, head back to the trail and follow it to the footbridge across the marsh. Turn right to follow the Mountain Dyke and have the binoculars ready to spot all the birdlife and beaver lodges. At the T-junction, head left, past the observation tower and onto Nature Dyke. Then just mosey along this idyllic treed pathway, taking in the sights and smells until you emerge at the narrows.

63 WIDGEON FALLS

Distance: 6 km	Rating: Easy
Elevation gain: Minimal	Season: Year-round
Hgh point: 25 m	Topographical map:
Time needed: 5 hours	Port Coquitlam 92G/7
(including paddling)	Trail map: Page 275

Note: You need a canoe or kayak to access the trailhead. Bring binoculars and an extra pair of shoes.

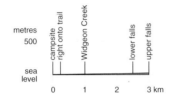

THE HIKE TO WIDGEON FALLS BEGINS WITH a lazy paddle up the quiet arms of Widgeon Slough through marshlands dotted with ducks, herons, hawks and many other varieties of birdlife. After that, it just gets even better.

To get to the starting point, take the Lougheed Highway to Pitt Meadows. Turn north on Dewdney Trunk Road, just after the Pitt River Bridge if you're coming from points west such as Vancouver, Burnaby and Coquitlam. At 208th Street (also known as Neaves Road), turn left. This later becomes Rannie Road; stay on it to Grant Narrows Regional Park.

If you don't bring your own canoe, you can rent one here. Ayla Canoe Rentals rents canoes by the day, but not every day. (Call 604–941–2822 for hours and rates.) Gord Williams and his Pitt Lake 'pit bull' (actually a toffee-coloured poodle who is mostly bark) can set you up with canoe, paddles and life jackets, and point you in the right direction.

Paddle across the narrows, keeping a watchful eye for power boats and jet skis. In late spring, look also for osprey, which nest on the pilings on the east side of Pitt River. Although osprey used to flourish throughout the Lower Mainland, Grant Narrows is one of the few sites where they are still known to nest.

Binoculars will be a big asset as you paddle through Widgeon Slough towards the campsite that marks the land-based portion of the hike. There are great blue herons fishing in the shallows, beaver lodges and gnawed sapling stumps nearby, and the occasional muskrat scooting for the cover of his hollow along the muddy banks.

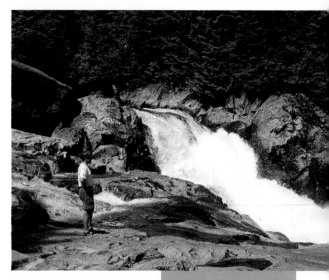

The slough is also unique in that it is a tidal freshwater wetland. The waters of Widgeon Slough, Pitt Lake and Pitt River rise and fall with the tides, despite the ocean's distance. You may get

Widgeon Falls has an upper and a lower section (seen here). Just watch your step: all the moisture here can mean slick spots.

first-hand experience of this phenomena if you paddle at low tide and have to pull your craft over exposed sandbars. For this reason, leave the hiking boots off until the campsite and wear sport sandals or old runners that you don't mind getting wet.

Geologically speaking, it wasn't long ago that Pitt Lake was part of the ocean. Thousands of years ago, before the Fraser River delta had become as built up as it is today with deposited silt and sediments, Pitt Lake was a saltwater fjord, much like Indian Arm is today.

Long before non-Natives arrived, this area was an important harvesting ground for the Katzie people. Food plants such as wapato (Indian potato), wild parsnips and wild carrots were gathered, and berries of all description were picked. The slough was also where cedar roots and strips were obtained for making baskets. Although the slough is not as plentiful today as it once was, says Katzie councillor Rick Bailey, Native Peoples still gather plants in the area for food and medicines.

All that history is something to consider once you get to the campsite and change your shoes. Then it's time to hike. Head north along an old gravel road in the direction of Widgeon

Creek. After a couple hundred metres, a sign marks the trail to the falls.

At first, the trail moves through a mixed forest of deciduous and coniferous trees. But not just the firs and cedars grow tall here. Many of the moss-covered maples top out the canopy at respectable heights of 20 to 30 metres.

Soon, any recent vandalism notwithstanding, you'll pass Chizzel the beaver, carved from a wooden post that makes up a foot bridge covering a boggy part of the trail. As the trail continues through the forest, look for Steller's jays flitting from branch to branch and red-tailed hawks soaring above. And on ground level, watch the path for toads and frogs.

At certain times of year, parts of the trail can be rather muddy. Non-slip, wooden platforms cross the boggiest portions, but you may have to glop through an occasional patch of muck. It's the perfect opportunity to look for animal tracks imprinted in the goo. Deer, bears, cougars and coyotes live in the area, as do foxes, minks and raccoons.

Eventually, the trail meets Widgeon Creek, then shadows it alongside a 10-metre cliff edge. The water in the pools seems preternaturally clear and green, like liquid emerald. The terrain becomes drier and the path strewn with fir needles. On the way are a few short steep sections—the only ones you'll encounter all day.

An hour or so after leaving the campsite, the trail leads to the lower falls with its clear swimming holes—perfect for a dip on a hot summer day; beautiful to look at on a cool fall afternoon.

Whatever the season, be careful. When wet, the rock can be slimy and slippery. One ill-placed step could mean a tumble into the frigid creek waters and a long, cold wet hike home.

To reach the upper falls, return to the main trail and continue another five to 10 minutes. This cascade is even more beautiful than the first. The rock has been sculpted by year after year of spring freshets, summer trickles and rain-swelled waters crashing down from Widgeon Lake—another 5 kilometres up the valley.

On a quiet fall day, it's a perfect perch for lunch, toe-soaking and peaceful reflection before heading back to civilization.

MAPLE RIDGE AREA

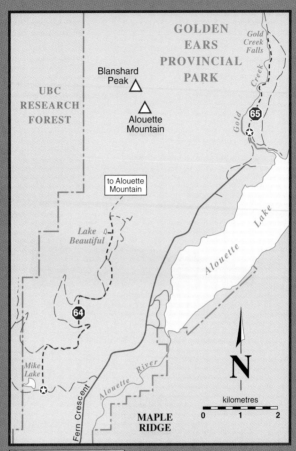

64 Alouette Ridge, p. 292
65 Gold Creek Falls, p. 296

64 ALOUETTE RIDGE

Distance: 14 km

Elevation gain: 550 m

High point: 800 m

Time needed: 5–6 hours

Rating: Moderate

Season: July to October

Topographical map:
  Port Coquitlam 92G/7 and
  Stave Lake 92G/8

Trail map: Page 291

Note: Dogs must be leashed.

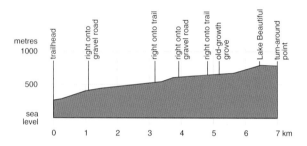

LOUETTE RIDGE HAS THE MISFORTUNE TO be plunked down next to some of the most magnificent mountain scenery in the Fraser Valley. The twin pinnacles of Golden Ears and the dramatic Blanshard Needle attract most people's attention, leaving Alouette Ridge an under-appreciated gem.

Less ostentatious glories—groves of lush old-growth forest, a tranquil water-lilied lake and a real feeling of being 'out there'—are the delights of Alouette Ridge. And although there may not be the same wow views as you get from the heights of Golden Ears, you also don't have a 10-hour slog involving 1500 metres of elevation gain.

Save Alouette Ridge for an overcast day, when its subtler beauty is best appreciated.

To get to the trailhead, first get to Golden Ears Provincial Park in Maple Ridge. Turn north off the Lougheed Highway onto 232nd Street and follow the blue and white BC Parks signs. Four kilometres from the park entrance and its 'can't-miss-it' giant mountain goat sign, turn left towards Mike Lake and the Park Headquarters. About 100 metres farther, stay left again, towards Mike Lake. Almost 2 kilometres distant is the start of the Incline Trail leading to Alouette Ridge. Park near the sign if possible, or 200 metres distant at the Mike Lake parking area.

The Incline Trail first crosses the outlet of Mike Lake, then comes to a junction. To the left is a 2-kilometre loop trail of

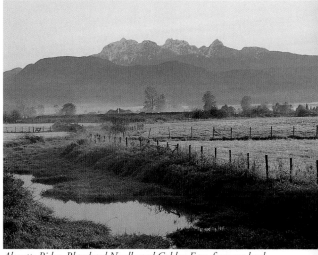

Alouette Ridge, Blanshard Needle and Golden Ears, from sea level.

Mike Lake. Stay right for now, and follow the old skid road through second-growth forest of western hemlock, western red cedar and Douglas fir, punctuated by big stumps and snags.

The trail climbs steadily then more steeply uphill, until about 15 minutes later it reaches the junction with the Eric Dunning Trail. A few minutes farther, the grade eases and the road joins with a fire access road. Stay right and follow the level road, stretching your leg muscles and catching your breath.

Soon, the road swings to the left, then crosses two nameless creeks. Not much farther past the second creek, the road makes a hairpin turn left. Fifty metres distant is an Alouette Mountain sign, noting a short-cut trail to the right. (You could continue on the fire access road for a more gradual climb, but it's almost three times as long.)

Here, the trail goes through more second-growth and more stumps. Although Golden Ears has been a provincial park since 1927, it wasn't declared a park until after vast swathes of the forest had been cut. The stumps here date from the 1920s when the Abernethy & Lougheed Company ran its logging operations. (One camp operated next to Mike Lake.)

At one time, the A&L operations were the largest in BC, employing more than 1000 men, 20 steam donkeys, seven steam locomotives, four boats and uncounted saws and axes to fell some of the biggest trees in coastal British Columbia.

More than 70 years later, the trees that have grown up in the place of the older giants now reach heights of about 15

> The trail continues through more old-growth with some truly monster snags, big beautiful trees and lush understorey. It's like a living museum of what once was all over Golden Ears Park—and the Lower Mainland.

to 20 metres and diameters of about 30 centimetres. By comparison, one of the biggest trees felled by A&L was a western red cedar that measured almost 3 metres in diameter.

About 20 minutes from its start, the short-cut trail greets the fire access road once again. Stay right and follow the level path to the only real viewpoint on the trail—across to Blue Mountain. If you hop the log and scoot down a few more metres you can also see Alouette Lake below and the snow-dusted top of Mount Crickmer. Just be careful, the unofficial path is slippery and overgrown.

Continue along the main path for another 10 minutes to the Alouette Mountain sign noting a trail branching right into the forest. If you've got a park map, you'll notice that the fire access road and this so-called short-cut trail look to be about the same length.

As you follow the trail through more second-growth and more stumps, you'll likely wonder why someone bothered to route a path through here. Then suddenly, the forest is transformed. The dark, spindly second-growth yields to a grove of lush old-growth forest with big trees and big snags of mostly western hemlock and western red cedar. The forest floor is no longer a lifeless brown mat, but a lush carpet of green moss, shrubs and tiny wildflowers.

In Golden Ears Park, where second-growth predominates on the trail, it's an unexpected, blissful surprise. Slow your pace to enjoy this little treasure and to ponder how A&L ever—happily—missed it.

All too soon, the trail emerges once again to the fire access road and a clearing. Go left to follow the Alouette Mountain and Lake Beautiful trail signs. (Just above the Lake Beautiful sign is a stately spiralling Douglas fir, topped but still growing strong.)

About 15 to 20 minutes in, the trail to Lake Beautiful branches left. Follow it down through a grove of big western cedars and along often-slippery boardwalk to the water's edge. Truth be told, it's more 'Pond Pretty' than 'Lake Beautiful,' with its small water-lilied surface and surrounding fringe of yellow cedar.

Regardless, it's definitely worth the effort to find a dryish perch and take a break, have some lunch and contemplate the tranquillity of the picture-perfect pondlet. You can also ponder the return trip. It's possible to continue farther up the main trail—all the way to Alouette Mountain, if you care to add another three to four hours to the trip. But it's a long, boggy way to get to any scenery worth the slog.

You may also notice on the park map that there is a trail about 15 to 20 minutes farther that connects the mountain trail to the fire access road. In reality, however, it is poorly marked and overgrown. The fire access road, although wide and clear at the start, also succumbs to dense foliage and becomes, at times, a very wet creekbed.

If you're into bushwhacking and have good routefinding skills, head up to the turnoff point. Look for a tangle of roots just past a small wooden footbridge; if you reach a long boggy stretch where you're forced to play hopscotch on embedded log sections, you've gone too far.

All in all, it's just as easy to retrace your steps from the lake to the clearing, once more through the marvellous grove of old-growth and down, down, down to the trailhead.

65 GOLD CREEK FALLS

Distance: 5.5 km	Rating: Easy
Elevation gain: Minimal	Season: Year-round
High point: 200 m	Topographical map:
Time needed: 2 hours	Stave Lake 92G/8
	Trail map: Page 291
Note: Dogs must be leashed.	

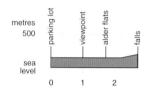

WHEN THE RAIN IS POURING DOWN, THE ground is more puddle than path and the temperatures are on the colder side of cool, you may still want to get out. You don't want it to be for a long time, just a good time; then back to hearth and home for a hot bath, a good book and a comfy chair. The perfect outing for this scenario is the Gold Creek Trail in Golden Ears Provincial Park.

A walk to the Lower Falls and back takes only two hours—even in the lousiest of weather. Should you have the fortune to do the walk on a clearer day, you'll find it to be among the prettiest places to stroll in the Lower Mainland.

To get to the trailhead, first get to Golden Ears Park in Maple Ridge. Turn off the Lougheed Highway and on to 232nd Street and continue north past Dewdney Trunk Road and follow the park signs. You're heading for the Gold Creek day-use area, about 14 kilometres from the park entrance with its giant mountain goat sign.

Once at the parking lot, head down one of the connecting paths towards the creek. And start following the trail, wide, obvious and leaf-covered, as it heads into classic West Coast rainforest. The trees within—trunks, branches and all—are attired in thick green sweaters of moss.

As you walk along, you'll notice massive erratic boulders, deposited thousands of years ago by some retreating glacier. Now, they're covered in moss and ferns and look like perfect miniature gardens.

Occasionally, you'll also see giant stumps, from formerly skyscraping cedar trees. In the 1920s, trees as large as 4 metres in diameter (as wide as a station wagon is long), met their fate

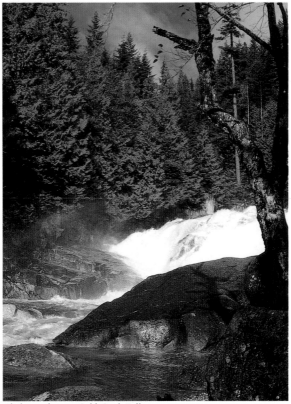

Slight rainbow at Gold Creek Falls.

under axe and crosscut saw. In 1931, a fire started here and raged through the valley, reducing most of the merchantable timber to ashes and bringing the Abernethy & Lougheed logging operations to an end. Fortunately, Douglas fir, western hemlock and red cedar have grown back, although not to the same epic proportions.

After 10 minutes of walking, you'll hear Gold Creek rushing just on the left. No need to leave the trail for a peek though; just a few minutes farther and you'll be walking alongside it. For the moment, as the trail undulates on gentle rises, just concentrate on the 'Emerald Forest' before you.

Where the trail dips past the 1-kilometre mark, the first views of the snow-frosted peaks to the north peek through. A little farther along, the vistas really open up. In winter and early spring, through the leafless branches of aspen and broadleaf maple trees, is a wide view of the narrow Gold Creek Valley tucked in between two mountain ridges.

On rainy days, the forest provides enough of a canopy to protect you from the droplets. When it's sunny, fingers of light reach through the overhead jungle and warm the forest and forest floor. Mist rises, and the rich, green scents of surrounding foliage deepen.

This valley and most other geographical features of Golden Ears Park were carved by vast ice sheets, which covered southwestern BC between 10,000 and 15,000 years ago. The sheets were so thick that most mountains were completely covered. Only the rocky summits of the highest park peaks—Mount Judge Howay at 2248 metres and Mount Robie Reid at 2087 metres—remained above ice.

Gold Creek Valley was likely formed when ice buildup on one of the nearby peaks trickled downslope in a tongue of ice, licking out a valley on the way. Meltwater traced new streams and carved deeper valleys as the ice receded and left deposits of finely ground soil and stone on the flatter sections.

Where the trail alongside Gold Creek flattens out, stop at one of the many gravel bars for a lingering look north at the peaks of Alouette, Blanshard and Edge mountains. In autumn, this area is popular with local photography buffs for its combinations of golden foliage, deep green conifers and snowy peaks.

Then, continue along the trail, scooting under a fallen alder and over a small wooden bridge into the forest again. For the next kilometre or so, the trail crosses several tumbling feeder creeks, via sometimes-slippery wooden bridges. And then, before you know it, you'll hear the roar and see the spray of the Lower Falls.

Soon, the tumbling falls themselves are visible. And as you get closer, you'll feel the spray. The view of the falls—a torrent of thick, white water that cascades about 25 metres—is well worth a wet face.

Follow the trail a couple of hundred metres farther to a higher, spray-free vantage point. From here, the water seems to tumble down a staircase of boulders into a deep pool of eddies and boils, before washing over the cliff edge. It's a mesmerizing, magnificent view, but don't be lured beyond the fenced area— it's slippery, steep and potentially dangerous.

Once you've absorbed enough spray, enough falls and enough tranquillity, head back down the trail, with all its views of mountain and forest, before returning home.

CHILLIWACK AREA

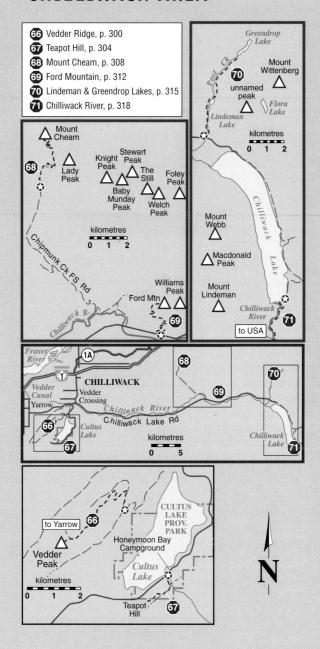

66 Vedder Ridge, p. 300
67 Teapot Hill, p. 304
68 Mount Cheam, p. 308
69 Ford Mountain, p. 312
70 Lindeman & Greendrop Lakes, p. 315
71 Chilliwack River, p. 318

Greendrop Lake

70 Mount Wittenberg

unnamed peak

Flora Lake

Lindeman Lake

kilometres
0 1 2

Mount Cheam

68 Knight Peak
Stewart Peak
The Still
Lady Peak
Foley Peak
Baby Munday Peak
Welch Peak

kilometres
0 1 2

Chipmunk Ck FS Rd

Chilliwack R.

Williams Peak
Ford Mtn
69

Mount Webb

Macdonald Peak

Mount Lindeman

Chilliwack Lake

Chilliwack River

71

to USA

Fraser River

1A

1

CHILLIWACK

Vedder Canal

Vedder Crossing

Yarrow

66

67

Cultus Lake

Chilliwack River

Chilliwack Lake Rd

68

69

70

Chilliwack Lake

71

kilometres
0 5

to Yarrow

66

CULTUS LAKE PROV. PARK

Honeymoon Bay Campground

Vedder Peak

Cultus Lake

kilometres
0 1 2

Teapot Hill

67

N

66 VEDDER RIDGE

Distance: 11.5 km	Rating: Moderate
Elevation gain: 375 m	Season: May to October
High point: 950 m	Topographical map:
Time needed: 4.5–5 hours	Mission 92G/1
	Trail map: Page 299

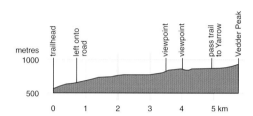

ALTHOUGH CLOSE TO CULTUS LAKE, THE trail to Vedder Ridge seems to exist in an entirely different universe than that of go-carts, power boats, waterslides and commercialization that characterizes the north end of the lake. Vedder Mountain Ridge Trail is a gentle pleasant hike through quiet mossy forest and sweet-scented glade with occasional views of all the lands surrounding and, at the top, a glimpse of the Pacific Ocean.

Vedder is probably best hiked in spring or fall when traffic isn't jamming Cultus Lake Road and the experience on top of Vedder Peak won't be marred by noise from below.

To get to the trailhead, follow Highway 1 east towards Chilliwack. Take exit #104 to Yarrow and follow the signs towards Cultus Lake. At Cultus Lake Road, turn right and zero the odometer.

At 2.2 kilometres, turn right onto Parmenter Road. At 2.8 kilometres, turn right onto Vedder Mountain Road. At 3.4 kilometres, turn left onto the Vedder Mountain Forest Service Road. At 6.5 kilometres, on the right of the road, a brown signpost notes the beginning of the Vedder Mountain Ridge Trail. Park well off the road in nearby pullouts.

Walk up an old jeep road for about 15 minutes to a junction. Go left to follow the signpost pointing the way to the trail and walk through second-growth forest. If it's rained recently, the air will be sweet with the scent of surrounding hemlock and fir, the trail shining with transcendent shafts of sunlight.

Where the road ends a few minutes later, the trail proper starts on the right as indicated by the signpost and map. Thanks for trail maintenance goes to the Valley Outdoor Association's

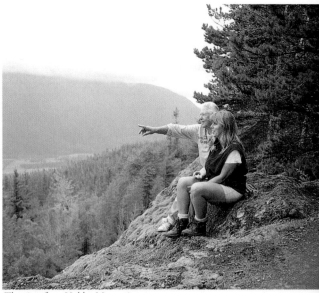

The view from Vedder Mountain.

Wednesday group.

A short, steepish ascent brings you a few minutes later to the 1.5 kilometre sign. The trail levels and wanders through a grove of older spruce, hemlock and Douglas fir, then rises gently to the 2-kilometre marker. Fifteen minutes or so later is the 2.5 kilometre marker (and just beyond a trail that cuts right to connect with Parmenter Forest Service Road).

Continue straight ahead to the 3-kilometre marker, a short, steep uphill grunt and then a longer steep grunt. Soon the 3.5-kilometre marker pops into view. Go right to a viewpoint of Sumas Prairie, Vedder Canal, Sumas Mountain and the Fraser Valley beyond.

The earliest mention of Sumas Mountain is found in Simon Fraser's 1808 journal of his epic Fraser River journey:

> Continued our course with a strong current for 9 miles where the river expands into a lake. Here we saw seals, a large river coming in on the left, and a round Mountain ahead, which the natives call shemotch... At this place the trees are remarkably large, cedars 5 fathoms in circumference and of proportional heights. Musketoes are in clouds and we had little or nothing to eat. The Natives always gave us plenty of provisions in their villages.

Shemotch, the Halkomelem name for Sumas Mountain,

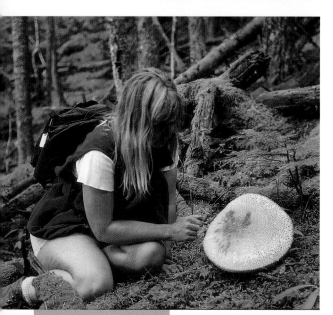

If you happen to be in the area in fall after a rainfall, you'll see mushrooms popping up all over. I once saw the biggest mushroom of my life here: it was the size of a pizza.

means 'gap left when a large chunk broke away' or 'divided head'—for the mountain's seemingly separate parts.

The name Sumas itself comes from 'Tuhk-kay-uqh,' a Halkomelem word meaning 'big flat opening.' Now this area is the Sumas Prairie, but once it was a lake 16 kilometres long and 10 kilometres wide, and good hunting grounds for the Native Peoples of the area.

Talk of claiming Sumas Lake began around the turn of the century. But it wasn't until 1919, at the urging of Chilliwack farmers, that Premier John Oliver authorized work to begin. Streams were diverted, dykes were built along the Vedder and Fraser Rivers and a drainage canal—the Vedder Canal—was built. The project, which had been estimated to cost $1.8 million, came in at more than $4.6 million. In 1922, the first house was built on the former lake.

After a restful water break, continue on the trail as it descends to a swampy section, then steadily climbs again and cross the ridge. About 15 minutes distant is one viewpoint, then another, with better views than the first.

Directly below is Cultus Lake, and across the valley is International Ridge. In the distance, part of the Chilliwack River valley is visible and, on a clear day, the ridge leading to Cheam Peak.

Trundle along for 15 minutes or so, then follow the trail as it descends to the 5-kilometre marker and a lakelet filled with water-lilies. The wooden bridges that carry you above the marshy muck surrounding the lakelet can often be slippery, so watch your footing.

Some western red cedars can be seen here. And lots of birds can be seen and heard.

Continue along the trail to a junction. Go left towards Vedder Peak. (Right goes to an old westside-trail from Yarrow.) For the next 15 to 20 minutes, the way is up, up, up as the trail regains the elevation it lost dipping down into the marshy area. Cross a slippery makeshift bridge and scramble up a rock bluff to eventually emerge to the peak and the 5.5 kilometre marker.

Vast views sprawl from the top, first of the Fraser Valley, then east to Cultus Lake. A short walk takes you to the true summit, where the views aren't as good but are still worthwhile. You can actually see the ocean.

The best places for lunch stops, though, are the viewpoints looking east. Gaze down to Cultus Lake, a popular summer spot.

The name 'Cultus' comes from 'kul,' a Chinook jargon word meaning anything bad, worthless or foul. The Sto:lo people believed that dreaded creatures called Seelkees lived in the lake. Seelkees were twice as big as a black bear but had legs like a beaver and a long tail. They often manifested themselves as dirty swirlings in the water. The actual Halkomelem name for the lake—'Swee-ehl-chah'—means 'unclear liquid that warns secretly.' Sweltzer, the anglicized form of the word, is now the name of the river draining the lake.

Once you've absorbed some of the tranquillity of Vedder Peak, retrace your steps to the forest service road.

67 TEAPOT HILL

Distance: 5 km	Rating: Easy
Elevation gain: 250 m	Season: Year-round
High point: 300 m	Topographical map:
Time needed: 2 hours	Chilliwack 92H/4
	Trail map: Page 299

Note: Dogs must be leashed.

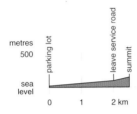

I N SOUTHWESTERN BC, THERE ARE SOME places that are only perfect for hiking or walking at certain times of the year, although they're accessible virtually year-round. One of those places is Cultus Lake Provincial Park. The perfect times to go are autumn, winter or spring, when the park is free of the speed boats, jet-skis and campers that swarm the lake in the summer.

For three seasons, the park is a haven of tranquil trails and sublime views of the surrounding peaks and ridges, with Cultus Lake itself like a smooth mirror reflecting the serenity of the so-called off-season.

Several trails, both for hikers and horseback riders, exist within the boundaries of the park. Most are short, and some, such as the loop trail to the Seven Sisters, lead to remnant big trees. Our destination is Teapot Hill: short, sweet and full of scenery with only a bit of elevation gain.

To get to the trailhead, follow Highway 1 east towards Chilliwack. Take exit #104 to Yarrow and follow the signs towards Cultus Lake. At Cultus Lake Road, turn right and follow the provincial park signs, eventually reaching the Columbia Valley Highway. Pass the waterslides and campgrounds to enter the park proper.

Drive past the campgrounds at Entrance Bay and Clear Creek. Another 500 metres will bring you within sight of the Teapot Hill trailhead parking lot. Head up the trail proper and within minutes, you'll come across a couple of metal park

A quiet creek and lush spring growth along the trail.

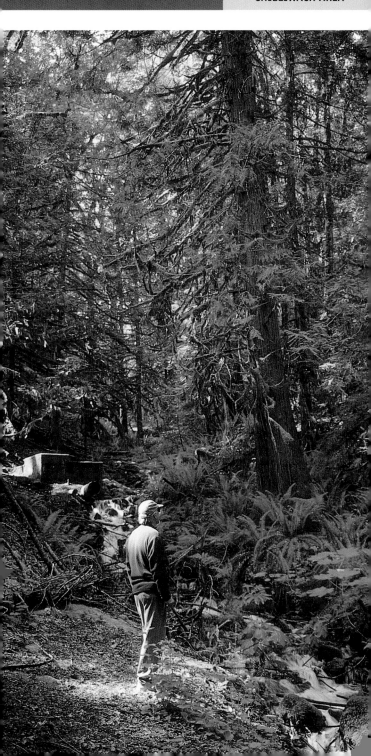

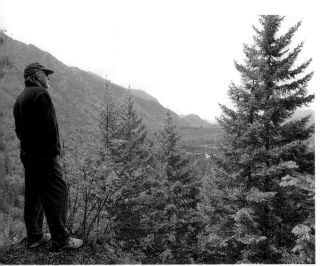

The view south to Columbia Valley.

signs, one with an area map and one that tells how Teapot Hill got its name.

In the 1850s, a couple of surveyors, it seems, followed an old deer trail to the top of the ridge, where they found a brass teapot. Whether it belonged to an early teetotalling logger, an old prospector passing through or some turn-of-the-century picnicker remains unknown.

Although the location of the Teapot Hill trail sign seems to indicate that you'd go off to the left here, **don't**. Instead, continue uphill along the service road, at times leaf-covered and needle-sprinkled. The trail winds gently upwards through groves of mixed deciduous and coniferous trees, and then the trail flattens out as it continues, about the same time as views of International Ridge, which flanks Cultus to the southeast, come into view. You may have to hop over an alder or two blown down by recent winds, but eventually you'll come to a point in the path where it's joined by a horse trail from the east.

Just stay on the service road and follow the little brown signs that point the way to Teapot Hill. Most of this means simply meandering dead ahead, but finally, after about 45 minutes or so, depending on your pace, you'll come to a point where you'll hang a right for the final jaunt to the top.

From here, the trail winds along the side of the hill. In just a few minutes, the trail crosses an invisible boundary from Cultus Lake Provincial Park to International Ridge Provincial Park. There's nothing to indicate the boundary—consider it a fun trivia fact.

At least 100 species of birds have been seen in the park over the years, including pileated woodpeckers and songbirds such as the red-eyed vireo (shown) and the black-throated grey warbler, not usually seen elsewhere in the Fraser Valley.

Soon, the trail emerges onto a bluff with two fabulous features—a lone Douglas fir, its top blown off, the length of its trunk scarred by a lightning strike, and Cultus Lake shimmering peacefully below.

In the mid-1800s, European settlers began to survey the land of the Chi-ihl-kway-uhk and Sto:lo peoples, staking out mining claims, homesteads and logging cutblocks. In 1859, Charles Wilson, secretary to Her Majesty's Boundary Commission, made this entry in his journal about a trip to Cultus Lake:

> The ride up the valley was very pleasant till we got to the lake; here we exchanged our horses for a boat, constructed by our men, and a very good one it was too and answered all the purposes wanted perfectly. The lake is about 3 miles long, the mountains coming straight down, the water beautifully clear and intensely cold like all other mountain lakes. You must bear in mind that when I talk about boats, trails, etc., they are nearly all of our own construction, as everything is in its wildest state here.

Walk past the Douglas fir to follow the path that bears left, for a second vast view—down the Columbia Valley to the US. Imagine what it must have looked like in its wildest state. Then, once you've absorbed enough of the surrounding serenity, head back down the path you came up on.

68 MOUNT CHEAM

Distance: 9.5 km	Rating: Moderate
Elevation gain: 630 m	Season: Mid-July to October
High point: 2112 m	Topographical map:
Time needed: 4 hours	Chilliwack 92H/4
	Trail map: Page 299

Note: A four-wheel drive vehicle is needed.

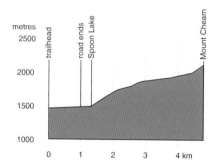

WILDFLOWER-FILLED MEADOWS AND stunning views are the only two reasons any hiker needs to head for the alpine. It's a hiker's dream come true when much of the upward slogging can be covered on road. Mount Cheam is such a destination.

To get to the trailhead, follow Highway 1 east to Chilliwack. Then follow the signs towards Chilliwack Lake Provincial Park. Eventually, they'll lead to the intersection known as Vedder Crossing. Turn south and follow the Chilliwack Lake Road as it shadows the Chilliwack River.

About 25 kilometres from Vedder Crossing, slow to look on the left for the Foley Creek Forest Service Road. Turn left and follow the road for about 2 kilometres, across Foley Creek. Go left. About 1.5 kilometres farther, turn right onto the Chipmunk Creek Forest Service Road and put your vehicle into four-wheel drive.

Continue to the fork at the 6-kilometre marker and stay right. Then, 2.3 kilometres farther, go right to follow the Mount Cheam signpost. Stay left at the next fork, 2.7 kilometres distant. Just a bit farther is the parking area.

Stop for a peek at the Mount Cheam signpost and trail, then start hoofing on the old logging road. Twenty minutes later, the road ends and a trail begins on the left, heading into lush alpine meadows. If you're here in autumn, look high on the

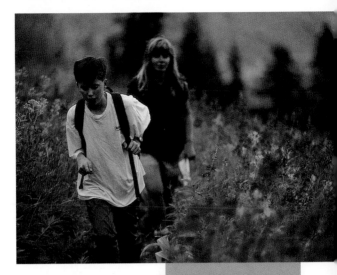

slopes and you may see black bears foraging for berries.

The name 'Cheam' comes from a Halkomelem word that means 'place to always get strawberries,' but that was what the Sto:lo people called a particular Fraser River island. The Native name for the peak is Thleethleq, after the protector of the Fraser River and spouse of Mount Baker.

Soon, the trail arrives at Spoon Lake, a sweet spot for a good long drink before starting the ascent.

The trail winds upwards through slopes drenched in wildflowers, even in late summer when other alpine meadows have faded. Bright pink fireweed, orange tiger lily, white Sitka valerian, yellow mountain arnica and a rainbow of other wildflowers line both sides of the trail and make the steady hike up more pleasant.

As the trail climbs, the views widen. Look south and it's one big clearcut—thousands and thousands of hectares worth. The view north is better: alpine meadows with groves of wizened subalpine fir, rife with blueberries and dotted with an occasional black bear. The trail switchbacks and traverses the slope at a steady uphill grade. About 30 minutes from Spoon Lake, the switchbacks steepen and cross to the north ridge.

Thick-girthed mountain hemlock can be seen here. And the occasional startled squeak of a pika can be heard as you near the ridgetop. Soon, the 2 kilometres pass and you're in a flattish

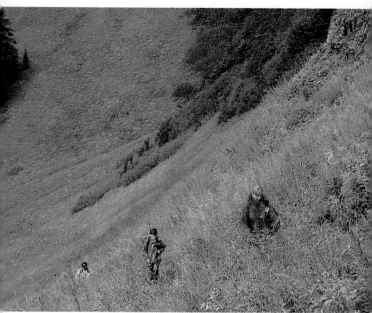

Fireweed in bloom along Mount Cheam Trail.

saddle. Take a break among the patches of alpine meadow and tiny seasonal tarns. (There's a short side-trail that leads to a precipitous view of Lady Peak's stunningly steep north face. Below are logging cutblocks and Jones Lake.)

From the saddle, the trail heads for the last 2.75 kilometres and 300 metres of elevation gain via a series of long, seemingly endless switchbacks. An hour should bring you to a junction with the old trail coming from Popkum way below. And, not much farther, is the summit itself.

The first ascent of Cheam was made in September 1888, from Popkum, by Misters Campbell, Knight, Thompson and two Native guides whose names were not recorded.

On a clear day at the top, the views are superb. To the west is the sprawl of Greater Vancouver with Georgia Strait in the distance. To the north are peaks such as Slollicum, Baird and the Old Settler. To the southeast are the peaks of the Cheam Range; among them are Stewart, Welch and Foley peaks and The Still, also known as the Lucky Four Group. Around World War I, miners built a trail up the creek leading to Welch and Foley to stake the Lucky Four Mine and prospect for copper.

It's all interesting history, but the best story of Cheam belongs to the first peoples of the area, the Sto:lo. According to Sto:lo legend, Thleethleq once accompanied Mount Baker to his country. There, they lived and raised three sons—Mount Hood, Mount Shasta and Mount Shuksan. Soon after, Thleethleq bore three daughters and announced her return to her people on the Sto:lo (the Native name for the Fraser River).

Once home, she and her daughters settled to watch over the people and the fish that return to feed them, so that no harm comes to either. According to Sto:lo elder Oliver Wells, now deceased, three small points on the mountain are Thleethleq's three daughters.

Sooner or later, you too will have to go back home. When you're ready, retrace your steps back to the vehicle.

69 FORD MOUNTAIN

Distance: 4.5 to 12.5 km	Season: June to October
Elevation gain: Up to 1000 m	Topographical map:
High point: 1420 m	Chilliwack 92H/4
Time needed: 2 to 5 hours	Trail map: Page 299
Rating: Moderate	

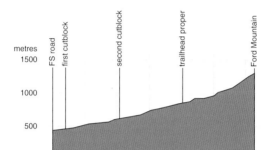

WHEN MOST PEOPLE THINK OF Chilliwack, they usually picture endless flat expanses criss-crossed by country roads and irrigation canals. Not many envision forested slopes, serrated granite peaks and glaciers, but it's all there in the Chilliwack Valley, along with an extensive network of hiking trails.

The peaks of the Chilliwack Valley are the northern end of the Cascades, the same mountain range in which you find the more well-known mounts of Baker, Rainier and St. Helen's. (The North Shore mountains and those of Squamish and Whistler belong to the Coast Range.)

Some peaks, like Mount Slesse, are classic North American mountaineering climbs, because of their height and technical difficulty. Others, like Mount Cheam and Ford Mountain, are easily accessed, hiker-friendly routes with fabulous views from the summit.

To get to the trailhead, follow Highway 1 east to Chilliwack. Then follow the signs towards Chilliwack Lake Provincial Park. Eventually they'll lead to the intersection known as Vedder Crossing. Turn south and follow the Chilliwack Lake Road as it shadows the Chilliwack River.

About 28.5 kilometres from the bridge at Vedder Crossing and just 2 kilometres after the road crosses to the north side of the river, slow down and look on the left side of the road for a brown sign noting the Ford Mountain Forest Service Road.

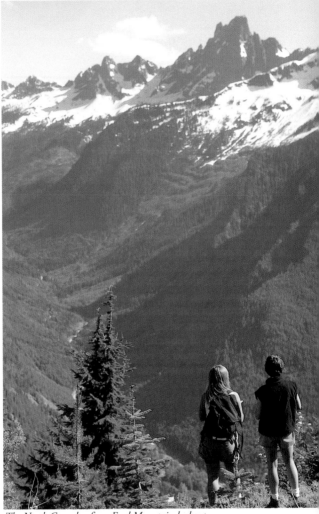

The North Cascades, from Ford Mountain lookout.

A four-wheel drive vehicle can make it up the first 4 kilo-metres of logging road, but you can also hike up. Drive as far as you can or want, and park in a wide pullout on the bump-and-grind road. (Most vehicles can make it up 750 metres to 1 kilometre of road.)

Cutblocks in various stages of regeneration stagger the road. If you hike the road in autumn, when berry bushes are thick and full, be sure to make noise as you walk, to warn any feasting black bears of your approach.

Filled with bright pink fireweed in summer or the muted colours of berry bushes in autumn, the road is a pleasant hike as it zigzags to the true trailhead.

All year-round, occasional glimpses through the trees hint at the views to come at the top. The distance between the first and second cutblock is about 1.75 kilometres, or 25 to 30 minutes of steady hiking. From the second cutblock to the true trailhead, it's another 2 kilometres, or 30 to 40 minutes of hiking.

The trail proper begins where a Chilliwack Forest District map points the way northeastward. At first, the trail winds steeply up. Go slow, following the orange diamond markers and occasional flutters of orange tape as the path gains elevation through the trees to the ridge.

After 20 to 30 minutes upward, the trail levels out and meanders through a sweet-scented hemlock grove. Twenty to 30 minutes more of such pleasant wandering brings you to the summit of Ford Mountain at 1421 metres. A forest service lookout stood here until the mid-1970s. Now all that remains are the concrete foundations, a few metal fragments and the views.

To the southeast is the shimmer of Chilliwack Lake. Directly east is Williams Peak, which pokes the sky at 1860 metres. The shining array of mountains to the north are the Lucky Four Group—the peaks of Foley, Welch, Stewart and The Still. The peaks are named after the partners in the mining firm of Foley, Welch and Stewart, which owned property in the area, most notably the Lucky Four Mine. The Still is so named for its resemblance to a bootlegger's spirit-making apparatus—vapour can occasionally be seen steaming from the gullies on the peak's north face. Look west to see far up the Chilliwack River valley.

To the south lies a horseshoe-shaped peak capped with ice—Mount Slesse. The name is derived from the Salish 'Sel-ee-see,' meaning 'fang.' The peak is famous both as a mountaineering marvel and as the site of a tragic 1956 air crash. In 1995, the BC government designated the mountain as a heritage site, thus creating a living monument to the 62 passengers and crew of TransCanada Airlines flight 810 who perished there. Beyond Slesse, out of sight, lies Mount Baker, a sleeping volcano that might once again spring to life as it last did in 1880.

Once you've rested your hiking legs and drunk in the views, return the way you came, knowing now that Chilliwack means 'mountains.'

LINDEMAN LAKE & GREENDROP LAKE

Distance: 4.5 to 10 km

Elevation gain: Up to 400 m

High point: 1000 m

Time needed: 2 to 5 hours

Rating: Easy to Lindeman; moderate to Greendrop

Season: June to October

Topographical map: Skagit River 92H/3

Trail map: Page 299

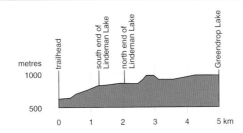

WHEN IT COMES TO LAKE DESTINATIONS, hikers usually favour two seasons—summer and fall. Summer lake-hikers look forward to a cool plunge at the end of a hot slog. Autumn lake-hikers are lured upward by the promise of fall foliage reflected in a surface of blue-green tranquillity.

The hike to Lindeman and Greendrop lakes can be a good summer hike, but it is best saved for autumn. The crowds of summer will have been washed away by the fall monsoons. Mosses, lichens and fungi will be growing luxuriantly on the forest floor. And the surrounding peaks will be dusted lightly with snow, the suggestion of winter yet to come.

To get to the trailhead, follow Highway 1 east to Chilliwack. Then follow the signs towards Chilliwack Lake Provincial Park. Eventually, they'll lead to Vedder Crossing. Turn south and follow the Chilliwack Lake Road as it shadows the Chilliwack River. Continue for about 38 kilometres to the Post Creek access road. If the road is barred, you'll need to park off the main forest service road and walk the final kilometre in. Otherwise, drive in to a small parking area and the trailhead.

After crossing the tiny bridge across Post Creek, look for the sign pointing the way to the lakes. At first, the trail winds upwards through an ancient boulder fall. Although the area was logged early in the 20th century, a couple of big, beautiful

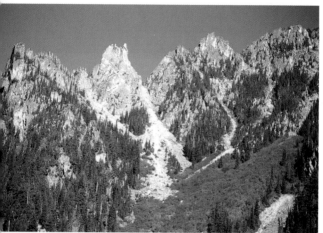

A view of the castellated peaks above Lindeman Lake.

Douglas firs remain anchored to the creekside slope. Pause for a look, then get ready to hike up, up, up for about 20 minutes.

Eventually, the trail levels, just past the point where crews have carved a couple of benches from downed snags. The 1-kilometre marker isn't much farther. A few minutes after that, the path enters the foot of a slide that tumbled long ago from the slope above. A few steps more and you're at the southern end of Lindeman Lake.

Lindeman Lake and Lindeman Peak (which lies near the US border and is not visible from here) were named after Chilliwack pioneer Harry Lindeman who reputedly used to carry fish up the trail to stock the lake.

The trail winds along Lindeman's western shore, opening up to views of long, scree slopes that, in season, are daubed with a palette of autumn colours—the golden leaves of slide alder, ochre-hued maples and crimson berry bushes—all reflected in incredibly clear turquoise waters. You'd be forgiven for thinking you'd suddenly been transported to the Canadian Rockies.

Where the trail crosses slopes of exposed rockfall, your footsteps will likely be accompanied by a chorus of distinctive *meep*s from the resident pikas. (For a look at these shy guinea-pig-sized rodents, you'll have to perch silently and motionlessly among the boulders.)

A few minutes after passing the 2-kilometre marker, the trail arrives at a soft sand beach on Lindeman's northern end. If you're content with a short hike for the day, this spot can be your lunch stop and turnaround point.

Many years ago, the Chi-ihl-kway-uhk people had some 30 villages along Chilliwack River. Trading routes went inland via Paleface Creek, Chum-chee hum (later Depot) Creek and this way, via Post Creek. In the mid-1800s, some of the trails were used by Hudson's Bay Company trappers. And more than 100 years later, the Post Creek route was included in the Centennial Trail, which stretches from Burnaby to Manning and Cathedral Lakes provincial parks.

> Between boulder fields, the trail dips into gullies of shimmering green mosses, flourishing second-growth cedar and fir, and a weird kaleidoscope of mushrooms, lichens and fungi. On some boulders grow what look like tiny, perfect Japanese gardens, as if cultivated by a bonsai master.

Save that epic for another time. If you're still up for another 6 kilometres and three hours of moderate hiking through boulder fields and sumptuous rainforest, continue along the trail towards Greendrop Lake. A word of caution: conditions at the higher lake can be as much as 10°C cooler than Lindeman, so be sure to take an extra fleece and other warm essentials.

As you follow the taped path north, the footing can be tricky, first while crossing a sometimes frost-covered boulder field, then while negotiating on and around slippery deadwood. Just remember, all that wetness has its benefits: namely the pockets of rain-drenched forest that lie ahead.

Within 30 minutes of leaving Lindeman is the 3-kilometre marker. And, if you don't dawdle too long, another half-hour will bring you to the 4-kilometre mark. Cross a couple of slippery log bridges over a tinkling low-water version of Post Creek, wander through the woods for another half hour or so and you'll come to Greendrop Lake.

Although not as scenic as Lindeman Lake, Greendrop has an ambiance all its own. Mist rises from the warm shallower waters at the south end, drifting up towards a waterfall tumbling down the lake's steep northwestern slope. After a well-earned break, retrace your steps to Lindeman and the Post Creek parking lot.

71 CHILLIWACK RIVER

Distance: 10.5 km	Season: April to October
Elevation gain: Minimal	Topographical map:
High point: 610 m	Skagit River 92H/3
Time needed: 3.5 hours	Trail map: Page 299
Rating: Easy	Note: Check road conditions first.

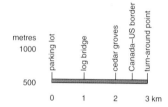

BEAUTIFUL VIRGIN FOREST FEATURING some of the biggest trees in southwestern BC is the undisputed highlight of a day-trip to the Upper Chilliwack River. But there are other attributes as well: secluded sandbars, mountain views and, in fall, spawning salmon.

To get to the trailhead, take Highway 1 east to Chilliwack, and then follow the signs towards Chilliwack Lake Provincial Park. At Vedder Crossing, turn south and follow the Chilliwack Lake Road as it shadows the Chilliwack River. About 28 kilometres in, the road changes from pavement to gravel. Another 12 kilometres brings the turnoff to the north end of Chilliwack Lake and the aforementioned park.

Continue straight ahead to follow a road that may be severely potholed or washed out. (You can check for conditions and closers by contacting the Chilliwack Forest Service Office. See information sources.) Stay right at any forks to arrive 9 kilometres later at Depot Creek. Park here.

Cross the bridge over Depot Creek and follow the old road for about two kilometres to reach the southern shore towards Chilliwack River. The name of the river and the lake, by the way, comes from a Halkomelem word meaning either 'quieter water on the head' or 'travel by way of a backwater or slough.'

Follow an unmarked trail through the brush and the trees. Watch all the time on the left for a lone Ecological Reserve sign, all that marks the start of the trail. You are in an eco-reserve, and you are not allowed to camp, fish or pick plants.

Follow the path into the forest and across a small, dilapidated wooden bridge. Almost immediately, you'll see big western red cedars and Douglas firs. The trail can be a bit overgrown here,

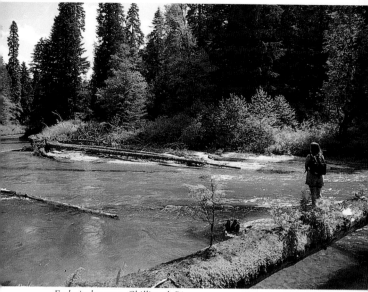

Ecological reserve, Chilliwack River.

but continue on. A few minutes farther is an 0.5 kilometre marker and another eco-reserve sign.

In 1980, 86 hectares of forest and marshland were set aside as Ecological Reserve No. 98 to protect the mature forest and the large western cedars and hybrid spruces contained within. Forests such as this were once common throughout the Lower Mainland, but 100 years of logging has left only pockets of old-growth trees at low elevations.

About 100 metres farther, the river appears once again and views of Middle Peak, just south of Mount Lindeman. Continue along the trail, lush in summer with ferns, salmonberry and the delicate white blooms of queen's cup, to the 1-kilometre marker. Cross a precariously tilted log bridge over a slough and you're back into the trees again.

Within 10 minutes, the trail enters a beautiful grove, which includes hybrid spruce trees believed to be a blend of coastal Sitka spruce and interior Engelmann spruce. At the base of one large specimen on the right, you can see faint markings of orange painted by researchers.

> Watch for a big amabilis fir, its lower limbs swaddled in lichen and giant bracket fungus. The tree is fit and straight but, at 400 years old, it is believed to be nearing the end of its lifespan.

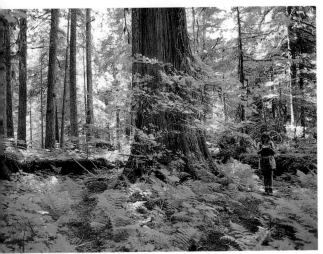

The 'monster tree.'

The trail continues through a remarkable grove of amabilis fir interspersed with western red cedar. Native Peoples chewed the pitch of amabilis fir (also known as balsam fir). Its sweet-scented boughs were used as bedding and floor-coverings in early Native households.

With almost all the trees pushing the 60-metre height, it may be a bit hard at first to pick out the 75-metre grand fir that is the biggest recorded specimen on record. Just look for the monster tree on the left of the path with its 3.6-metre diameter trunk nestled in devil's club. (For comparison, it's worth noting that this tree stands as tall as the downtown Vancouver Block building with its distinctive clock.)

Ten to 15 minutes farther, the trail enters another beautiful cedar grove. Soon after is the 2-kilometre marker, and not much farther, another big grove of cedar.

As you pass the 2.5 kilometre sign and emerge from the trees, you will be able to see the trough, cut into the treed slopes high above, which marks the US border. A few metres farther is a signpost noting the beginning of the North Cascades National Park and the regulations for anyone wanting to camp in its backcountry. (For information, call 360-599-2714.)

On the ground is another sign with 'Free Southern Cascadia' written on it by some wag. The trail beyond here is rougher, more overgrown and less frequently trodden than that on the Canadian side, but it's worth trekking a bit farther to find an empty sandbar on which to have lunch, relax and enjoy one of the last great forests in the Greater Vancouver area.

SKAGIT VALLEY & MANNING PARKS

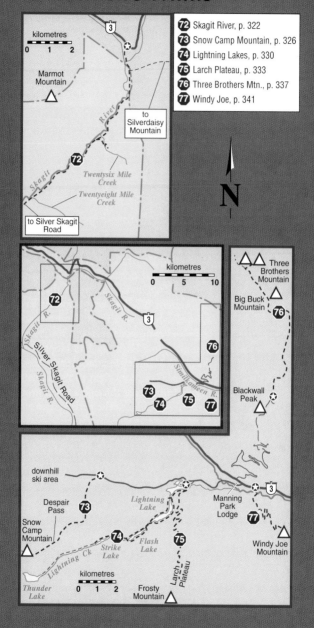

N

kilometres
0 1 2

Marmot Mountain

Skagit River

to Silverdaisy Mountain

72

Twentysix Mile Creek

Twentyeight Mile Creek

to Silver Skagit Road

kilometres
0 5 10

Skagit R.

Skagit R.

Silver Skagit Road

Skagit R.

72

73

74

75

76

77

Similkameen R.

Three Brothers Mountain

Big Buck Mountain **76**

Blackwall Peak

downhill ski area

Despair Pass

Snow Camp Mountain

73

Lightning Lake

Lightning Ck

Strike Lake

74

Flash Lake

75

Larch Plateau

Manning Park Lodge

77

Windy Joe Mountain

Thunder Lake

kilometres
0 1 2

Frosty Mountain

72 SKAGIT RIVER

Distance: Up to 20 km	Rating: Moderate
Elevation gain: Minimal	Season: May to October
High point: 650 m	Topographical map:
Time needed: Up to 7 hours	Skagit River 92H/3
	Trail map: Page 321

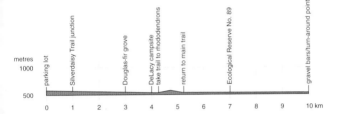

ONCE A ROUTE FROM BELLINGHAM TO THE
fur-bearing and mineral riches of the BC Interior,
the Skagit River Trail today is one of the most
pleasant hikes in southwestern BC. The way is mostly level
and leads past abandoned cabins, wild rhododendrons and
groves of stunning cedar and cottonwoods.

To get to the trailhead, follow Highway 1 to Hope, then
head east along Highway 3 to Manning Provincial Park. About
10 kilometres past the West Gate, turn right to the Sumallo
Grove picnic area. A gravel road leads through a lovely grove
of Douglas fir and western red cedar to the parking area and
the trailhead.

Before hitting the trail, take a moment to read the BC Parks
signboard, which notes that the Skagit River Trail was once part
of the Whatcom Trail, built in 1858 to provide access from the
US to Hudson's Bay Company brigade trails in the BC Interior
and the goldfields of the Fraser Canyon.

The route was less than a roaring success, however, as the
man charged with its construction, US Engineer Captain
Walter DeLacy, dragged it across three 2000-metre-high
mountains. Two months after its official opening, the 430-
kilometre trail was abandoned.

From the parking area, follow the trail leading to the left
along the river and cross the bridge. The trail follows an old
road through a copse of alder and cottonwood. Twenty minutes
later is the intersection with the Silverdaisy Trail.

About 100 metres farther, an unmarked trail on the left
veers off for an interesting side-trip to a waterfall, an old mine

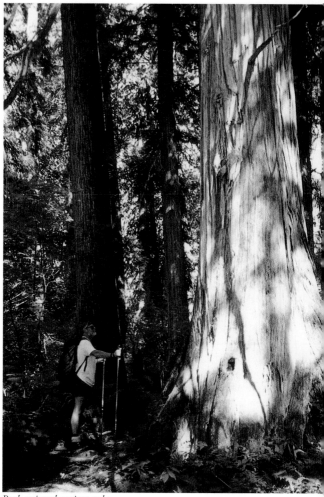

Bark-stripped ancient cedar.

entrance and decrepit cabin. The rusted hulk of an old Ford truck marks the spot. A clue to the age of the vehicle can be found in the dashboard panel—the speedometer only goes as high as 60 mph.

Retrace your steps to the main trail. Soon, the trail passes a 2-kilometre marker, then 15 minutes later a grove of beautiful old Douglas firs. Watch your step when looking up; you wouldn't want to land in the devil's club that lines both sides of the trail. The Skagit River runs alongside, making for a distinctly sylvan setting.

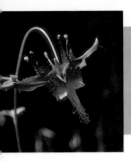

Along the way, the trail is lined with wildflowers—tiny blue forget-me-nots, fragrant wild rose and lily-like columbines (shown), called 'red rainflowers' by the Haida.

The name 'Skagit' comes from the Coast Salish people who lived along the river. Its relevance is not entirely clear, but the name is believed to have come from a Salish word meaning 'to hide or conceal.'

The 4-kilometre marker passes 20 to 25 minutes later. Not much farther is DeLacy Camp, a somewhat dark place to pitch an overnight tent, but with great views of some big western red cedars, some of whose roots have been exposed where the river has undercut the bank.

A few minutes farther, just when you first hear the sound of Twentysix Mile Creek ahead, a footpath branches to the left, marked by orange flagging tape and blue-blazed trees. In June and July, it's a side-trip worth making to see the groves of wild rhododendrons. A 15-minute foray brings you to the heart of the grove, but the trail winds higher and higher upslope if you just can't get enough of the delicate pink blooms.

Retrace your steps to the main trail and continue south to Twentysix Mile Creek. After crossing the creek, the trail wanders through a lush forest of ferns, huckleberry and large western red cedars. Twenty minutes later, the 5-kilometre marker appears.

The trail continues wandering along the river, rising at times to rocky bluffs. Eventually, at kilometre 6, a sign notes the northern boundary of Ecological Reserve No. 89. In 1978, 69 hectares of forest floodplain were set aside to protect the cottonwood stands along the Skagit River, but it's the exquisite western red cedars that will grab your attention first.

As the trail wanders the flats, it passes several magnificent trees, some 10 metres in girth and 60 metres high—about as tall as the old Sun Tower in downtown Vancouver. The late Randy Stoltmann, in his posthumously published book *Hiking the Ancient Forests of British Columbia and Washington,* notes that bark-stripping scars are visible on some of the cedars. The bark, he says, may have been used to build temporary fishing shelters.

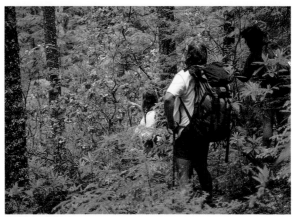

Wild rhododendron grove.

The trail also passes black cottonwoods that rival the cedars in height. The cottonwoods' heart-shaped leaves turn yellow in autumn—an awesome sight. This spot is a suitable turnaround point if your hiking day will be fulfilled by the time you retrace the previous 6 kilometres.

In summer, though, it's worth going farther south through a younger fire-scarred forest of Douglas fir and western hemlock, over talus slopes and through another beauty grove of western red cedar to eventually cross Twentyeight Mile Creek via log.

Just beyond is the 9-kilometre marker and gravel bars that are the perfect place to stop for lunch and a well-deserved break. You might even include a dip in the chill of the river. (The trail continues for another 5.5 kilometres to emerge on the Silver Skagit Road, 45 kilometres southeast of Hope, but you've seen the best scenery already.)

Looking south from the gravel bars, you should be able to catch a glimpse of the 2294-metre Whitworth Peak, also within the new Skagit Valley Provincial Park.

Just out of sight, to the south is Shawatum Mountain, known to early pioneers as Steamboat or Lost Musket Mountain. In 1910, a couple of fun guys reported finding gold on the slopes of Shawatum. A brief stampede of gold-seekers hit the old Whatcom Trail. By the time the hoax was uncovered, more than 1200 mining claims had been staked and the townsite of Steamboat built, complete with stores and a hotel.

When you've finished lunching, swimming, sunning or catnapping, retrace your steps to the parking area at Sumallo Grove.

73 SNOW CAMP MOUNTAIN

Distance: 17 km	Season: July to October
Elevation gain: 600 m	Topographical map:
High point: 1980 m	Manning Park 92H/2
Time needed: 6 hours	Trail map: Page 321
Rating: Moderate	

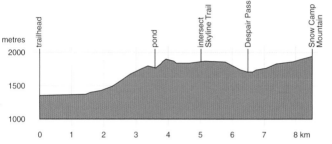

SOME HIKERS SHUN PROVINCIAL PARKS FOR

wilder, less-known terrain. The trails are too trammelled, they say, the people too numerous. And sometimes, they're right.

But every once in a while there is a path that reminds us how glorious parks can be. Take Manning Provincial Park, for example. As the second-most popular park in the province, it attracts about 1.5 million people to day-use areas in a single year, with another 114,000 people camping at the park's four campgrounds.

Sure, it means overflowing parking lots and picnic tables at Lightning Lakes. And sure, the Heather Trail—where you can drive to the alpine—attracts swarms of hikers. But where a little effort is involved, fewer folks are to be found. The hike to Snow Camp Mountain often attracts fewer hikers.

To get to the trailhead, turn off Highway 3 at Manning Park Lodge and follow the road past the stables toward the Lightning Lakes day-use area. Take the right fork past the campground, toward Gibsons Pass ski area. Park at Strawberry Flats, where the yellow gate bars the road.

Turn right at the big mapboard and follow the wide gravel path to the junction with Three Falls Trail. Then bear left to take the narrower track through the open field and into the forest. Ten minutes later is the 1-kilometre marker and the beginning of the day's ascent. A lush understorey of foamflower, fern and huckleberry bush supports a forest that contains trees that are surprisingly big, given the elevation—almost 1500

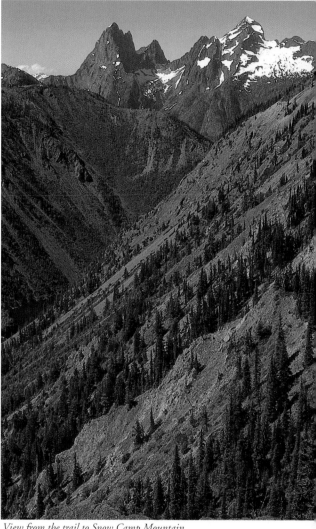

View from the trail to Snow Camp Mountain.

metres—and severe conditions in which they grow.

Steadily but gradually, the trail climbs. After crossing a small creek, the 2-kilometre marker appears, then 15 minutes or so later, the 3-kilometre marker. Ten minutes later, the trail begins to level out and emerges into a subalpine meadow coloured with pale yellow western anemones, bright yellow buttercups and deep blue lupines.

After passing the 4-kilometre marker and a small swampy

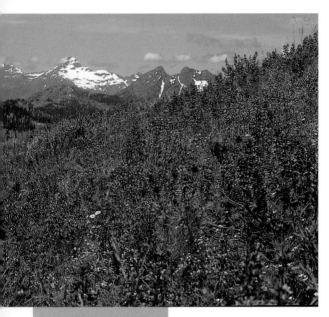

For a moderate amount of upward effort, the rewards include killer views of Hozameen Mountain and other peaks of the North Cascades, and virtual carpets of alpine wildflowers.

pond, the trail heads upward again, through an old burn. Despite the 50 years that have passed since the forest fire, the forest has been slow in coming back, thanks to the shorter growing season and higher elevation. The young green trees are still overpowered by the fire remnants; some snags stand bleached white by the sun, while others are still charred black.

While the cool of the forest has been temporarily lost, open views of Manning's eastern portions have been gained. In the distance, it's possible to see the road that snakes to the Cascade Lookout and Blackwall Peak. Farther behind are subalpine meadows, through which the Heather Trails winds, and the first peak of the Three Brothers Mountain.

As the trail continues back into the trees, traversing a ridge top, the elevation gain abates. At the 5-kilometre marker, the trail emerges to the first big views of the day. The aptly named Red Mountain lies directly across the valley, while Snow Camp Mountain (our destination), Lone Goat and the surrealistic Hozameen Mountain dominate the view to the southwest.

The double-summit, 2500-metre peak is actually located in the United States, where it's spelled 'Hozomeen.' In the Thompson language, 'Hozameen' means 'sharp, like a sharp knife.' The peak was first climbed in 1904.

As the views open up, the wildflowers increase in abundance—Indian paintbrush, mountain arnica and tiger lily. The trail dips down, then emerges at the junction with the Skyline Trail that comes from Lightning Lakes (a longer, stiffer approach). On this side of the ridge, the slope sheers steeply into the valley below. Looking east, you can just spot Strike Lake. Looking west, you can make out part of remote Thunder Lake.

Long before fur traders and gold seekers plied the routes through what is now Manning Provincial Park, the trails were used extensively by Native Peoples. Coastal Natives travelled inland along what is now the Skyline Trail. They carried dried salmon and oolichan to trade for the red ochre gleaned by Interior bands at what was once called Vermillion Forks (now Princeton).

Native people living in the Similkameen Valley used to climb the same mountain ridges in search of berries and marmots, whose soft coats were used in making winterwear.

After a well-deserved break, follow the trail right and down into Despair Pass. The 6-kilometre sign zips past in a blur, but by the 7-kilometre mark, you'll start to understand how the pass got its name. On a hot day, it seems like a long slog up, up, up. In reality, it's 30 to 40 minutes of moderate switchbacks and open meadows to the alpine with its profusion of wildflowers and endless mountain views.

Where a rock slide crosses the trail, you can look 750 metres straight down to where Thunder Lake sparkles like a sapphire. The trail continues another 1.5 kilometres to Lone Goat Mountain or 3 kilometres to Camp Mowich, but we'll make this spot the turnaround point.

If you want to make it to the actual summit of Snow Camp, there is a rough route that leads up. Just remember, these are extremely fragile meadows, so either stick to the already-trodden ground or find a spot just off-trail to enjoy the flowers, views and one of the best hikes in southwestern BC.

74 LIGHTNING LAKES

Distance: 14 km

Elevation gain: Minimal

High point: 1250 m

Time needed: 4.5–5 hours

Rating: Easy to moderate

Season: May to October

Topographical map:
    Manning 92H/2

Trail map: Page 321

Note: Dogs must be leashed.

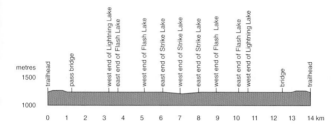

ONCE THEY WERE CALLED THE QUARTET Lakes, but some more creative soul must have been sparked by the beauty of the place—or perhaps was caught out in an electrical storm—because now the lakes have their more descriptive and deserving monikers of Lightning, Flash, Strike and Thunder.

Most of the 1.5 million people who visit the day-use areas in Manning Provincial Park come here, but many of them never go farther than the beach. And of those people who do venture onto the lake trails, most go no farther than the end of the first section of the first lake—Lightning.

What a shame. The lake trails are the perfect destination for any level of hiker. The ground is level, the scenery increasingly beautiful as you head farther from the picnic grounds, and the day can last as long as you want. It's even great when it's raining. (During one particular downpour, I talked my dad into hiking all the way to Strike Lake. We only turned around because we were hungry and looking forward to a hot lunch at the park restaurant.)

The route we'll follow covers about 14 kilometres and takes 4.5 to 5 hours return, but it's possible to do shorter loops or a longer, eight-hour epic hike.

To get to the trailhead, follow Highway 1 to Hope, then take Highway 3 east to Manning Park Lodge. Turn right on the Lightning Lakes Road and follow it past the stables. Where the road forks, bear left to the day-use area.

From the parking lot, walk along the lakefront to the

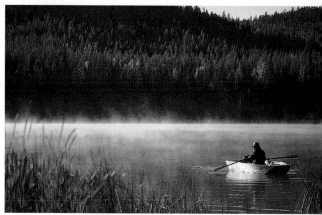

Mist over Lightning Lake.

easternmost end of the lake. Turn right and cross the bridge over Little Muddy Creek. The embankment on which you're walking is a dam.

Before 1966, the part of Lightning Lake that sees most of Manning Park's visitors was a marsh. When the creek was dammed, the marshland was flooded. *Et voilà*, a new lake.

At the end of the dyke, where the trail to Frosty Mountain heads uphill, stay right and along the lakeshore. As the trail meanders along the south shore, the way is lined with lodgepole pine, Engelmann spruce and some Douglas fir, all draped with long strands of witch's hair lichen. There are views across to Skyline Trail, and even on a rainy day, you can see determined fishermen bobbing along in belly boats hoping for a nibble.

Eventually, the Rainbow Bridge crosses the water-filled channel between the two sections of Lightning Lake. If you wanted only a one-hour walk, you could cross and head back to the day-use area. Instead, check out the view from the span, then continue along the south shore of the original Lightning Lake.

About 25 metres distant, look down from the trail to the water's edge to see a beaver lodge. Then continue along. In summer, a few wildflowers can be seen along the trail. And in fall, mushrooms pop out all over the forest floor. Because fewer people make the trip farther than the Rainbow Bridge, the forest and lake here have a quieter, wilder feel.

About 25 minutes from the bridge, the trail traverses a rock fall and, 10 minutes farther, crosses Frosty Creek to come to a beautiful clearing filled with big trees and big devil's club. Not much farther, the trail leads to the end of Lightning Lake. What looked to me like a jumble of old concrete bricks and

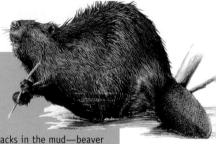

Where the trail passes under the unmistakable bushy green track of an avalanche chute, wander down to the lakeshore. You'll likely see animals tracks in the mud—beaver (shown), muskrat, deer, maybe even black bear.

old logs are in fact, says my fisherman dad, remnants of an old fish ladder.

At the trail junction, you could go right and follow the signs to the day-use area for a three-hour return trip, but we'll go left and continue on to Flash Lake.

A few minutes later, the trail splits. Go left and downhill, across the wooden bridge into a grove filled with thimbleberry, mountain ash, devil's club, Engelmann spruce and lodgepole pine.

The trail soon emerges to views of a vast marsh at the east end of Flash Lake, home to beaver, deer, bear and the occasional moose. Evidence of beaver can be seen in the dams, the gnawed saplings along the trail and the Taj Mahal of beaver lodges in the open marsh.

On the south shore of Flash, hikers get to see what the lakes were like before all the crowds. The trail on which you're hiking was originally an old trapping trail. Beaver, mink and otter, with their rich furs, were the prized prey of early 20th-century trappers.

Here, where the slopes are steep, it's easy to see how the lakes were once an ancient channel left behind by receding glaciers. The lakes, it is believed, were formed when the slopes eroded and the resulting debris blocked the meltwater.

As the trail nears the end of Flash, it passes through a beautiful grove of western red cedar and Engelmann spruce. Cross over Middle Creek and follow the split log planks to the lodge bridge at the western end of flash.

At the trail junction, you can go right and along the north shores of Flash and Lightning lakes to the day-use area. Alternatively, you could turn left and explore 1 kilometre farther to the beginning of Strike Lake, which is more marsh than lake, or 5 kilometres farther to the most distant lake—Thunder.

Whichever choice you make, be sure to leave enough time to get back to the day-use area.

LARCH PLATEAU 75

Distance: 18 km	Season: July to October
Elevation gain: 800 m	Topographical map:
High point: 2000 m	Manning Park 92H/2
Time needed: 7 hours	Trail map: Page 321
Rating: Moderate	Note: Dogs must be leashed.

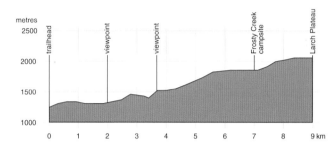

THERE ARE AT LEAST TWO KINDS OF HIKERS in the world. First, there are those who live by the motto 'Another week, another peak,' and are not satisfied unless an outing delivers another summit to bag. Second, there are those for whom the journey is just as important as the destination.

And it is to those latter hikers that we dedicate this trip. On the journey, you will find wildflowers and lichen-drenched forest, grand views and subalpine meadows. The destination is equally spectacular—the largest stand of alpine larch in south-western BC and, quite possibly, the oldest trees in Canada.

To get to the trailhead, follow Highway 1 to Hope, then take Highway 3 east to Manning Park Lodge. Turn right on the Lightning Lakes Road, follow it past the stables and, where the road forks, bear left to the day-use area.

From the parking lot, wander down to the shore of Lightning Lake, then head east and over the bridge that crosses an outlet creek. The embankment on which you're walking is a dam. Before the dam was built, the lake in front of you was essentially a marsh.

On the far shore, look for the signposted trail to Frosty Mountain and follow it up. (Yes, even BC Parks is part of the mountain-summit-as-destination conspiracy.) The trail makes a gradual ascent via a long switchbacking traverse. Bright yellow mountain arnica, deep blue lupines and pristine white

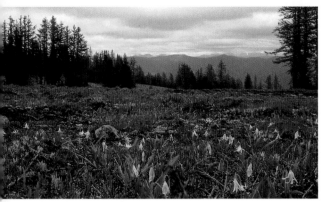

Glacier lilies, Larch Plateau.

bunchberry line the trail. The forest is mostly lodgepole pine and Engelmann spruce supported by a lush understorey.

About 20 minutes up, the trail passes the 1-kilometre marker and then more wildflowers: red columbine, queen's cup, foamflower, Sitka valerian. Fifteen minutes farther is a viewpoint that looks out over Lightning and Flash lakes. The triangular point of Red Mountain peeks from the northwest.

A few minutes farther brings the 2-kilometre sign. Soon after, the trail levels a bit, passing through more patches of wildflowers: tiger lilies, showy locoweed, Indian paintbrush, lance-leaved stonecrop.

Thirty minutes later of wandering upwards on this lovely trail brings you to more views, not only of the lakes below but also of peaks, such as jagged Hozameen Mountain, which form the backdrop to the Skyline Trail. A virtual wash of flowers covers the slopes here: you're essentially walking through a subalpine meadow, albeit one at a 45° angle.

Another few minutes brings another viewpoint, then the trail crosses to the east side of the ridge. After 20 minutes steady uphill, the trail finally levels to a plateau filled with higher-elevation wildflowers: lupine, creeping phlox and the unmistakable mop-tops of western anemones gone to seed, also known as tow-head babies.

The trail rambles pleasantly south through forest and meadow, each replete with its own particular garden of flowers, for about 25 minutes to eventually pass the 'Wilderness Camp 1 km' sign. Sure enough, 10 minutes later is the campsite at Frosty Creek. An old cabin inhabits the site, but only desperation and certain immunity to the hanta virus would make me sleep within.

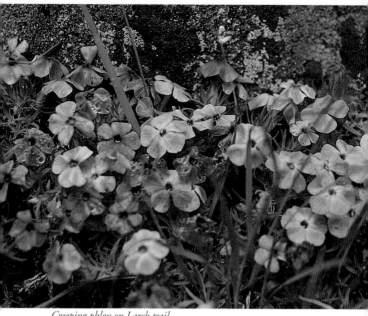

Creeping phlox on Larch trail.

Cross Frosty Creek and head upslope, zigging and zagging your way to a viewpoint only 15 minutes distant. To the west is Frosty Mountain in all its steep, icy splendour. The true summit of Frosty at 2423 metres, is right before you. (But don't tell that to all the hikers who think they've got to the top when they've really just made it to the second-highest of Frosty's summits. It'd make 'em crazy.)

Be sure to take the switchback here that swings left (an old trail continues straight ahead to a big rockslide). Within minutes, the first of the alpine larch appears, as does white heather. Ten minutes farther, views to the northeast open up. And just a bit farther is the 8-kilo-metre marker.

Soon after, you enter a wide, open plateau treed almost exclusively by alpine larch—also called woolly larch, tamarack, Lyall larch

Larch are conifers, but they're unusual in that they're the only conifer to shed their needles in winter. Alpine larch is an especially hardy species, existing in places that are too cold for other trees. Its soft, green needles push out in spring and, in autumn, turn a blazing gold.

and subalpine larch. Its species name, *Larix lyalli*, honours the Scottish surgeon and naturalist David Lyall, who first described the species in 1858.

Although alpine larch is common in more easterly parts of BC such as the Selkirk, Purcell and Rocky mountains, it's comparatively unusual in this neck of the woods. (Another species of larch, western larch, grows at lower elevations and is more commonly seen.)

Because of the short growing season, thin soil and harsh conditions of the alpine, most alpine larch grow no higher than 25 metres and no fatter than about 60 centimetres—about the same size as a plumpish lamppost.

These particular alpine larch are believed to be more than 2000 years old, based on projections of growth rates from the outer rings of rotted older trees. There is talk of setting the plateau aside as an ecological reserve within the park.

Mountain goats, bighorn sheep, black and grizzly bears all feed in alpine larch stands. But you don't have to worry about such company here: only black bears inhabit the southern portion of Manning Park and they're probably busy noshing on roots or berries lower down.

So, find a good spot within view of a particularly lovely cluster of alpine larch and feed on lunch yourself. Afterwards, you can wander farther up the plateau to the height of land, even to the trail junction, where peak-baggers face an additional three hours of up and down. There is also another trail, which heads northeast to emerge on the Windy Joe Trail. But it's a longer, less interesting return than simply retracing your steps to Lightning Lake.

THREE BROTHERS MOUNTAIN 76

Distance: 22 km	Rating: Strenuous
Elevation gain: 400 m	Season: July to September
High point: 2272 m	Topographical map:
Time needed: 7–8 hours	Manning Park 92H/2
	Trail map: Page 321

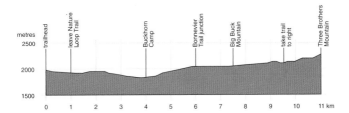

MOST HIKES THAT INVOLVE THE BEAUTY of alpine meadows and high-elevation views require a long slog up. On some hikes, such as the way to Three Brothers Mountain, most of the ascent is done in a vehicle on a road.

Although some people might consider it cheating, the fact is the length of this hike still means a good long workout. So ignore the purists and let them start from the bottom if they want.

The only drawback to having such easy access to the alpine is that a lot of other people are also drawn to the hike. In summer, the parking lot at Blackwall Peak is often jammed and the trails crowded. An abundance of wildflowers can help take your mind off hiker overload, but then there's the bugs—no-see-ums, blackflies and deer flies—that can make me run screaming for the vehicle.

To my mind, early autumn is the best time to enjoy the alpine leading to Three Brothers. Meadows smoulder in hues of gold and ochre, scarlet and mauve. And most of the bugs and the crowds have gone.

To get to the trailhead, first get to the Manning Park Lodge in Manning Provincial Park. Turn north to follow the steep and winding road—about 6 kilometres of pavement to Cascade Lookout, then another 5 or so kilometres of gravel road to the parking lot at Blackwall Peak.

Although most of the rock that underlies Manning Park is sedimentary, giving clues to the ancient sea that once covered the area, Blackwall Peak is an exception. It's believed the now-

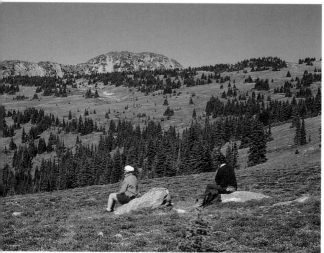

View from Big Buck Mountain.

rounded peak is the remnant part of a volcanic cinder cone, composed of basalt (crystallized lava).

The Heather Trail leaves from both the lower and upper lots. Choose the upper, with its eastward views; follow the Nature Loop Trail over a small rise then down into the heather. Soon after is, appropriately, the Heather Trail. Go straight to follow its gentle descent into a timbered valley.

When I last did the route, I was fortunate enough to meet Rob Christie, an environmental forester who interpreted the surrounding forest for me, pointing out the advanced age of baby-sized spruce, and reading the area's forest fire history through its burnt snags and more recent growth.

By the time we reached Buckhorn Camp, the trees felt like family, with Rob as the family genealogist/historian weaving tales of generations present and past. (For similar information, drop in at the park's information centre where exhibits and wardens can provide some insights into the natural history of the area.)

As you pass through the designated campsite, notice the several regeneration projects in progress. The subalpine environment is fragile and can take decades to recover from such simple damage as that done by hikers going off trail. Parks staff have covered and cordoned off the worst areas, to help the meadows to recover.

Heading out of camp, the trail begins a long, slow wind through cool coniferous groves and open burned sites, gaining in elevation to the open sub-alpine meadows of Big Buck Mountain (and the junction with the Bonnevier Trail).

On a topographical map, Big Buck looks more like a big plateau than a mountain. The resulting 360° views from here make it easy to see why the area has been a popular destination since early in the 20th century.

The closest peaks are Windy Joe and Frosty mountains, both within the boundaries of the park; most of the distant peaks are over the border, in the US. To the east is the drier Okanagan Range, its mountains thick with trees. To the west are the snow-capped mountains of the northern Cascades, with the stiletto peaks of the Hozameen Range and the glacier-topped Silvertip Mountain most prominent.

> Between 1913 and 1930, the wilderness area was popular for guide-led packhorse trips. Evidence of even longer use has been found at Buckhorn Camp in the blazes that mark some of the spruce trees along the stream below the shelter. One such blaze dates to 1876, the oldest visible date on park record, and is presumed to have been cut by a passing prospector.

To the north is the continuing trail. If you decide to continue farther, follow the trail through meadows, over tiny trickling creeks and across rocky ravines to a saddle overlooking the vast green expanse of the Copper Creek watershed.

It was in this area that the first non-Native—Paul Johnson—set up a trapline in the early 1900s. In 1906, Johnson sold his trapping rights to a couple of Americans now known only as Levitt and Ryder. They trapped the Three Brothers area for two years and pretty much depleted the fur-bearing population. After having trapped out the line, the duo sold their interests to brothers Harry and Bill Gordon, who trapped the area in a less devastating manner for three decades.

Then, early in 1931, the Three Brothers Mountain Reserve was set aside, primarily to save the alpine meadows from over-grazing by domestic sheep. Five years later, part of it was included in a new game reserve. And in 1941, the Ernest C. Manning Provincial Park (commonly referred to simply as Manning Park) was created, named after the province's chief forester who had recently died in a plane accident.

From here, drop down into the saddle, then follow the trail up for a few hundred metres to a junction with the route to the top of the first Brother. This summit is the first of the three that make up Three Brothers Mountain. The way is steep and

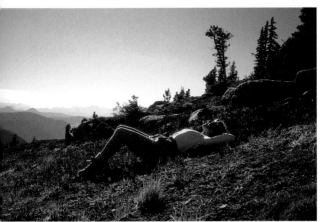

Relaxing admidst fall meadow foliage.

rocky, at one point traversing a skinny ridge where both sides sheer dramatically away to the valleys below.

If you're uncomfortable with heights or queasy at the thought of scrambling on hand and foot to a high place, leave the summit for another time when you're feeling up to such a challenge. You might pause to consider that at one time these peaks were even steeper and more stiletto-like than today. A vast ice sheet during the last glaciation, between 10,000 and 15,000 years ago, scraped over the Three Brothers and rounded its summits.

If you do make it to the top, be prepared for the cold winds. You'll probably want to spend only enough time to drink in the views and grab a photo with the summit sign, before descending and retracing your many steps back to the parking lot.

WINDY JOE

77

Distance: 15 km	Rating: Moderate
Elevation gain: 525 m	Season: June to October
High point: 1825 m	Topographical map:
Time needed: 4–5 hours	Manning 92H/2
	Trail map: Page 321

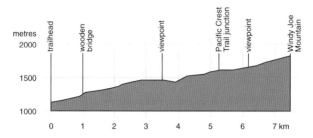

POOR WINDY JOE. SURROUNDED AS HE IS BY the magnificence of his alpine siblings, most people don't even notice his lushly forested presence on the south side of the highway. But anyone who thinks of Joe as a lacklustre hiking destination makes a big mistake. The hike to Windy Joe has big views and one of the only remaining forest fire lookouts in the province, and it requires only modest amounts of time and effort.

It's best done as part of a weekend getaway, but it's still possible as a city-based day-hike. Just keep in mind that Windy Joe is at least three hours drive from Vancouver each way.

Either Manning Park Lodge area or the Beaver Pond parking lot can be used as the trailhead. We start where the trail begins just on the eastern edge of the Manning Park Corral. (Look for the brown signpost noting the way to Beaver Pond.)

A wide flat trail runs along the north bank of the Similkameen River through a mixed forest of big cottonwoods, spruce and lodgepole pine. Fifteen to 20 minutes of walking brings you to a trail junction. Straight uphill goes to the highway; the lower trail leads to Beaver Pond. We'll go right, over the old wooden bridge following the signs to Windy Joe.

(If you come from Beaver Pond, just follow the signs west for about 10 minutes to the same trail junction.)

A few minutes farther, a steel and wood truss bridge crosses a larger fork of the Similkameen. About 75 metres farther is a T-junction. Left leads to Castle Creek. We'll go right, hot on the trail of Windy Joe.

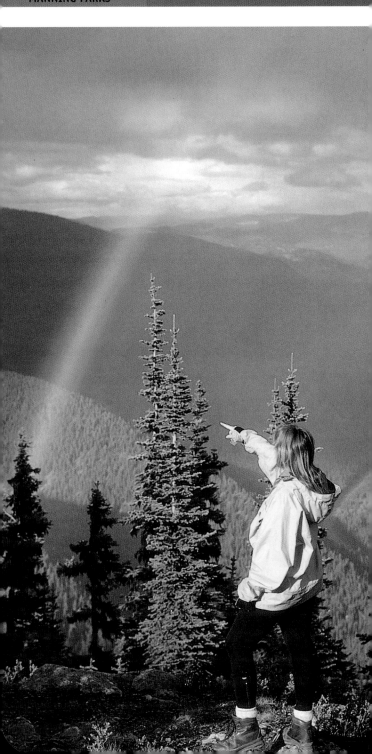

Not long after is the red 1-kilometre marker. From here, the old access road climbs gradually and steadily to the top through a forest that sighs and creaks with each breath of wind. Strands of wire still hanging from the trees are all that remain of the communication system that was used by lookout rangers to alert parks staff in the valley to forest fires.

The 2-kilometre marker flashes by about 15 to 20 minutes after you passed the first. Just a few minutes farther, the tinkle of a nameless creek below accompanies this section of the trail. A bit farther, the old road crosses the same creek. And a bit farther still is the 3-kilometre marker.

Some big, thick, tall, lichen-draped interior firs can be seen growing in the gully below. Although they may not be as big as some of the coastal giants, they're equally impressive for having reached this size at this elevation.

The old road recrosses the creek twice more, and in a few minutes is a viewpoint that looks to the northwest, up Gibson Pass Road to forested hills beyond. Before you know it, the 4-kilometre marker is passed. About 10 minutes farther the trail splits. The way south heads to Frosty Mountain and the entire 4200 kilometres of the Pacific Crest Trail, which travels through Washington, Oregon and California right to the Mexican border.

Save that hike for another time (it would take about 40 days), and continue left, reaching the 5-kilometre marker in another few minutes. Just beyond a big off-trail boulder, look on the right side of the trail for an old pre-metric trailmarker nailed to a tree.

Before you know it, the 6-kilometre marker is passed, then another viewpoint, then the 7-kilometre marker and *voilà*, the summit of Windy Joe at 1825 metres.

The mountain is named after Joe Hilton, who worked in the park from 1946 to 1975. As the story goes, Hilton's old trapping partner thought of the name in reference to his buddy's constant remarks on how the winds here were so strong they kept the summit clear of snow in winter. (Maybe in the old days that was true, but one winter when I snowshoed to the top there was lots of white stuff—and frostbite temperatures.)

The first rangers on Windy Joe spotted fires from a tent. In 1950, the lookout tower was built. It was used for 13 years until airplanes became the standard for fire-spotting.

Panoramic panels painted above show what you're looking at out there. To the south is Monument 83, Ptarmigan Peak and Mount Winthrop. To the southeast are more peaks of the

Rainbow over Windy Joe Summit.

On the top floor of the lookout is an old firefinder. When a ranger spotted distant smoke, he'd determine the position of the blaze by lining up the sights of the finder with the smoke, then relay the information to Park Headquarters in the valley below.

Cascade Range, which at less than 10 million years old is one of the youngest mountain ranges in the world.

To the west is Castle Peak in the US, Frosty Mountain and the distinctly sawtoothed outline of Frosty Ridge. Although Frosty at 2408 metres is the highest peak in Manning Park, it's estimated that its peak protruded only 250 metres above the thick glaciers that covered the area between 10,000 and 15,000 years ago during the last ice age.

To the northwest are Shawatum and Silver Tip mountains; to the north are Mounts Outram, Ford and Dewdney; and to the northeast is Blackwall Peak and Three Brothers Mountain.

It's a lot to take in, so remember to bring a lunch—and in cooler months a warm fleece or wool sweater, a toque and gloves—to linger and dote on Windy Joe. When you're finished doting, retrace your steps to the start.

HIKES BY DURATION

TWO HOURS

Brunswick Point: 2 hours
Cougar Mountain: 2–3 hours
Cypress Falls: 2 hours
Dog Mountain: 2 hours
Gold Creek Falls: 2 hours
Killarney Lake: 2–3 hours
Lighthouse Park: 2 hours
Point Grey Foreshore: 2–5 hours
Seymour River & Rice Lake
    Loop: 2 hours
Stanley Park: 2 hours
Teapot Hill: 2 hours

THREE HOURS

Capilano Canyon: 3 hours
Cheakamus Canyon: 3 hours
Chilliwack River: 3.5 hours
Hollyburn Ridge: 3 hours
Lynn Canyon & Seymour River
    Loop: Up to 3 hours
Lynn Creek & Forest Loop:
    3–4 hours
Minnekhada: 3 hours
Pacific Spirit Regional Park:
    Up to 3 hours
Stawamus Chief: South
    Summit: 3–4 hours

FOUR HOURS

Alice Lake Provincial Park:
    Up to 4 hours
Baden-Powell: Lynn Canyon
    to Grouse Mountain:
    4–5 hours
Brandywine Meadows:
    3–4 hours
Brothers Creek Loop: 4 hours
Buntzen Lake: 4 hours
Mount Cheam: 4 hours
Hollyburn Peak: 4 hours
Lightning Lakes: 4 hours
Lynn Peak: 4 hours
Shannon Falls: 4 hours

FIVE HOURS

Alouette Ridge: 5–6 hours
Baden-Powell: Deep Cove
    to Lynn Canyon: 5 hours
Baden-Powell: Cleveland Dam
    to Cypress Bowl: 5 hours
Black Mountain: 5 hours
Black Tusk: 5 hours
Blowdown Pass: 5 hours
Cheakamus Lake: 5 hours
Ford Mountain: Up to 5 hours
Goat Mountain & Ridge:
    4–5 hours
High Falls Creek: 4–5 hours
Howe Sound Bluffs: 5 hours
Joffre Lakes: 5 hours
Levette Lake Loop: 5 hours
Lindeman & Greendrop Lakes:
    Up to 5 hours
Mosquito Creek Cascades:
    Up to 5 hours
Norvan Falls: 5–6 hours
Opal Cone: 5 hours
Panorama Ridge: 5 hours
Petgill Lake: 5–6 hours
Pitt Wildlife Loop:
    Up to 5 hours
Mount Seymour: 5–6 hours
St. Mark's Summit: 5 hours
Stawamus Chief: Centre &
    North Summits: 5 hours
Tenquille Lake: 5 hours
Vedder Ridge: 4.5–5 hours
Widgeon Falls: 5 hours
Windy Joe: 4–5 hours

SIX HOURS

Mount Artaban: 6 hours
Baden-Powell: Cypress Bowl to Eagle Ridge: 6 hours
Sendero Diez Vistas: 6 hours
Elfin Lakes: 6 hours
Mount Gardner: 5 hours
Garibaldi Lake: 6 hours
Munro & Dennett Lakes: 6 hours
Rainbow Lake: 6 hours
Skagit River: 6–7 hours
Snow Camp Mountain: 6 hours
Stawamus Squaw: 6 hours
Mount Strachan: 6 hours

SEVEN HOURS+

Deeks Lake: 7 hours
Eagle Ridge: 6.5–7 hours
Hanes Valley: 6–7 hours
Larch Plateau: 7 hours
The Lions: 6–7 hours
Russet Lake: 10 hours
Three Brothers Mountain: 7–8 hours
Wedgemount Lake: 7–8 hours

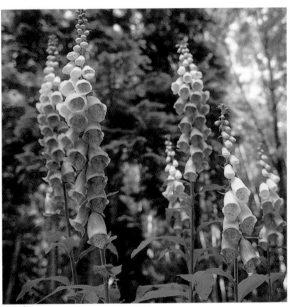

Foxgloves.

HIKES BY DIFFICULTY

EASY HIKES (24)

Alice Lake Provincial Park
Baden-Powell: Deep Cove
    to Lynn Canyon
Brunswick Point
Capilano Canyon
Cheakamus Canyon
Cheakamus Lake
Chilliwack River
Cypress Falls
Dog Mountain
Gold Creek Falls
Hollyburn Ridge
Killarney Lake
Levette Lake Loop
Lighthouse Park
Lynn Canyon &
    Seymour River Loop
Lynn Creek & Forest Loop
Minnekhada
Pacific Spirit Regional Park
Point Grey Foreshore
Seymour River &
    Rice Lake Loop
Stanley Park
Teapot Hill
Widgeon Falls

MODERATE HIKES (45)

Alouette Ridge
Mount Artaban
Baden-Powell: Lynn Canyon
    to Grouse Mountain
Baden-Powell: Cleveland Dam
    to Cypress Bowl
Baden-Powell: Cypress Bowl
    to Eagle Ridge
Black Mountain
Blowdown Lake & Pass
Brandywine Meadows
Brothers Creek Loop
Buntzen Lake
Mount Cheam
Sendero Diez Vistas

Elfin Lakes
Ford Mountain
Mount Gardner
Garibaldi Lake
Goat Mountain & Ridge
High Falls Creek
Hollyburn Peak
Howe Sound Bluffs
Joffre Lakes
Larch Plateau
Lightning Lakes
Lindeman & Greendrop Lakes
Lynn Peak
Mosquito Creek Cascades
Munro & Dennett Lakes
Norvan Falls
Opal Cone
Panorama Ridge
Petgill Lake
Pitt Wildlife Loop
Rainbow Lake
Mount Seymour
Shannon Falls
Skagit River
Snow Camp Mountain
St. Mark's Summit
Stawamus Chief: South Summit
Stawamus Chief:
    Centre & North Summits
Stawamus Squaw
Mount Strachan
Tenquille Lake
Vedder Ridge
Windy Joe

STRENUOUS HIKES (8)

Black Tusk
Deeks Lake
Eagle Ridge
Hanes Valley
The Lions
Russet Lake
Three Brothers Mountain
Wedgemount Lake

HIKES BY MONTH

ALPHABETICAL

	J	F	M	A	M	J	J	A	S	O	N	D
Alice Lake	x	x	x	x	x	x	x	x	x	x	x	x
Alouette Ridge							x	x	x	x		
Artaban, Mount	x	x	x	x	x	x	x	x	x	x	x	x
Baden-Powell Trail: Deep Cove to Lynn Canyon	x	x	x	x	x	x	x	x	x	x	x	x
Baden-Powell Trail: Lynn Canyon to Grouse	x	x	x	x	x	x	x	x	x	x	x	x
Baden-Powell Trail: Cleveland to Cypress						x	x	x	x	x		
Baden-Powell Trail: Cypress to Eagle Ridge							x	x	x	x		
Black Mountain						x	x	x	x	x		
Black Tusk							x	x	x	x		
Blowdown Pass							x	x	x			
Brandywine Meadows							x	x	x	x		
Brothers Creek			x	x	x	x	x	x	x	x	x	
Brunswick Point	x	x	x	x	x	x	x	x	x	x	x	x
Buntzen Lake	x	x	x	x	x	x	x	x	x	x	x	x
Capilano Canyon	x	x	x	x	x	x	x	x	x	x	x	x
Cheakamus Canyon		x	x	x	x	x	x	x	x	x	x	
Cheakamus Lake			x	x	x	x	x	x	x			
Cheam, Mount							x	x	x	x		
Chilliwack River		x	x	x	x	x	x	x				
Cougar Mountain			x	x	x	x	x	x				
Cypress Falls	x	x	x	x	x	x	x	x	x	x	x	x
Deeks Lake							x	x	x	x		
Dog Mountain						x	x	x	x	x		
Eagle Ridge						x	x	x	x	x		
Elfin Lakes							x	x	x	x		
Ford Mountain						x	x	x	x	x		
Gardner, Mount	x	x	x	x	x	x	x	x	x	x	x	x

	J	F	M	A	M	J	J	A	S	O	N	D
Garibaldi Lake							x	x	x	x		
Goat Mountain							x	x	x	x		
Gold Creek Falls	x	x	x	x	x	x	x	x	x	x	x	x
Hanes Valley							x	x	x			
High Falls Creek				x	x	x	x	x	x			
Hollyburn Peak							x	x	x	x		
Hollyburn Ridge					x	x	x	x	x			
Howe Sound Bluffs				x	x	x	x	x	x			
Joffre Lakes							x	x	x			
Killarney Lake	x	x	x	x	x	x	x	x	x	x	x	x
Larch Plateau							x	x	x	x		
Levette Lake Loop			x	x	x	x	x	x	x			
Lighthouse Park	x	x	x	x	x	x	x	x	x	x	x	x
Lightning Lakes					x	x	x	x	x			
Lindeman & Greendrop Lakes						x	x	x	x			
The Lions							x	x	x	x		
Lynn Canyon & Seymour	x	x	x	x	x	x	x	x	x	x	x	x
Lynn Creek & Forest Loop	x	x	x	x	x	x	x	x	x	x	x	x
Lynn Peak				x	x	x	x	x	x	x		
Minnekhada	x	x	x	x	x	x	x	x	x	x	x	x
Mosquito Creek			x	x	x	x	x	x	x	x		
Munro & Dennett Lakes					x	x	x	x	x			
Norvan Falls	x	x	x	x	x	x	x	x	x	x	x	x
Opal Cone							x	x	x			
Pacific Spirit	x	x	x	x	x	x	x	x	x	x	x	x
Panorama Ridge						x	x	x	x			
Petgill Lake			x	x	x	x	x	x	x	x		
Pitt Wildlife Loop	x	x	x	x	x	x	x	x	x	x	x	x
Point Grey Foreshore	x	x	x	x	x	x	x	x	x	x	x	x
Rainbow Lake							x	x	x	x		
Russet Lake							x	x	x	x		
St. Mark's Summit						x	x	x	x			

	J	F	M	A	M	J	J	A	S	O	N	D
Sendero Diez Vistas			x	x	x	x	x	x	x	x		
Seymour, Mount						x	x	x	x			
Seymour River & Rice Lake	x	x	x	x	x	x	x	x	x	x	x	x
Shannon Falls			x	x	x	x	x	x	x	x	x	
Skagit River			x	x	x	x	x	x	x			
Snow Camp Mountain						x	x	x	x			
Stanley Park	x	x	x	x	x	x	x	x	x	x	x	x
Stawamus Chief: South		x	x	x	x	x	x	x	x	x		
Stawamus Chief: Centre & North		x	x	x	x	x	x	x	x	x		
Stawamus Squaw		x	x	x	x	x	x	x	x	x		
Strachan, Mount						x	x	x	x			
Teapot Hill	x	x	x	x	x	x	x	x	x	x	x	x
Tenquille Lake							x	x	x	x		
Three Brothers Mountain						x	x	x	x			
Vedder Ridge				x	x	x	x	x	x			
Wedgemount Lake						x	x	x				
Widgeon Falls	x	x	x	x	x	x	x	x	x	x	x	x
Windy Joe							x	x	x	x		

HIKING SEASONS: SHORTEST TO LONGEST

	J	F	M	A	M	J	J	A	S	O	N	D
Blowdown Pass						x	x	x				
Hanes Valley							x	x	x			
Joffre Lakes						x	x	x				
Opal Cone						x	x	x				
Wedgemount Lake						x	x	x				
Alouette Ridge						x	x	x	x			
Baden-Powell Trail: Cypress to Eagle Ridge						x	x	x	x			
Black Tusk						x	x	x	x			
Brandywine Meadows						x	x	x	x			
Cheam, Mount						x	x	x	x			
Deeks Lake						x	x	x	x			
Elfin Lakes						x	x	x	x			
Garibaldi Lake						x	x	x	x			
Goat Mountain						x	x	x	x			
Hollyburn Peak						x	x	x	x			
Larch Plateau						x	x	x	x			
The Lions						x	x	x	x			
Panorama Ridge						x	x	x	x			
Rainbow Lake						x	x	x	x			
Russet Lake						x	x	x	x			
Seymour, Mount						x	x	x	x			
Snow Camp Mountain						x	x	x	x			
St. Mark's Summit						x	x	x	x			
Strachan, Mount						x	x	x	x			
Tenquille Lake						x	x	x	x			
Three Brothers Mountain						x	x	x	x			
Windy Joe						x	x	x	x			
Baden-Powell Trail: Cleveland to Cypress					x	x	x	x	x			
Black Mountain					x	x	x	x	x			
Dog Mountain					x	x	x	x	x			

	J	F	M	A	M	J	J	A	S	O	N	D
Eagle Ridge					x	x	x	x	x			
Ford Mountain					x	x	x	x	x			
Hollyburn Ridge					x	x	x	x	x			
Lindeman & Greendrop Lakes				x	x	x	x	x				
Munro & Dennett Lakes				x	x	x	x	x				
Cougar Mountain					x	x	x	x	x	x		
High Falls Creek					x	x	x	x	x	x		
Howe Sound Bluffs					x	x	x	x	x	x		
Lightning Lakes					x	x	x	x	x	x		
Vedder Ridge					x	x	x	x	x	x		
Chilliwack River			x	x	x	x	x	x	x			
Cheakamus Lake			x	x	x	x	x	x	x			
Lynn Peak			x	x	x	x	x	x	x			
Skagit River			x	x	x	x	x	x	x			
Levette Lake		x	x	x	x	x	x	x	x			
Sendero Diez Vistas		x	x	x	x	x	x	x	x			
Brothers Creek			x	x	x	x	x	x	x	x	x	
Mosquito Creek			x	x	x	x	x	x	x	x	x	
Petgill Lake			x	x	x	x	x	x	x	x	x	
Shannon Falls			x	x	x	x	x	x	x	x	x	
Stawamus Chief: South			x	x	x	x	x	x	x	x	x	
Stawamus Chief: Centre & North		x	x	x	x	x	x	x	x	x		
Stawamus Squaw		x	x	x	x	x	x	x	x	x		
Cheakamus Canyon		x	x	x	x	x	x	x	x	x	x	
Alice Lake	x	x	x	x	x	x	x	x	x	x	x	x
Artaban, Mount	x	x	x	x	x	x	x	x	x	x	x	x
Baden-Powell Trail: Deep Cove to Lynn Canyon	x	x	x	x	x	x	x	x	x	x	x	x
Baden-Powell Trail: Lynn Canyon to Grouse	x	x	x	x	x	x	x	x	x	x	x	x
Brunswick Point	x	x	x	x	x	x	x	x	x	x	x	x
Buntzen Lake	x	x	x	x	x	x	x	x	x	x	x	x

	J	F	M	A	M	J	J	A	S	O	N	D
Capilano Canyon	x	x	x	x	x	x	x	x	x	x	x	x
Cypress Falls	x	x	x	x	x	x	x	x	x	x	x	x
Gardner, Mount	x	x	x	x	x	x	x	x	x	x	x	x
Gold Creek Falls	x	x	x	x	x	x	x	x	x	x	x	x
Killarney Lake	x	x	x	x	x	x	x	x	x	x	x	x
Lighthouse Park	x	x	x	x	x	x	x	x	x	x	x	x
Lynn Canyon & Seymour	x	x	x	x	x	x	x	x	x	x	x	x
Lynn Creek & Forest Loop	x	x	x	x	x	x	x	x	x	x	x	x
Minnekhada	x	x	x	x	x	x	x	x	x	x	x	x
Norvan Falls	x	x	x	x	x	x	x	x	x	x	x	x
Pacific Spirit	x	x	x	x	x	x	x	x	x	x	x	x
Pitt Wildlife Loop	x	x	x	x	x	x	x	x	x	x	x	x
Point Grey Foreshore	x	x	x	x	x	x	x	x	x	x	x	x
Seymour River & Rice Lake	x	x	x	x	x	x	x	x	x	x	x	x
Stanley Park	x	x	x	x	x	x	x	x	x	x	x	x
Teapot Hill	x	x	x	x	x	x	x	x	x	x	x	x
Widgeon Falls	x	x	x	x	x	x	x	x	x	x	x	x

SELECTED BIBLIOGRAPHY

Akrigg, Philip and Akrigg, Helen. *British Columbia Place Names*. Victoria: Sono Nis, 1986.

Armstrong, John. *Vancouver Geology*. Vancouver: Geological Association of Canada, Cordilleran Section, 1990.

Beckey, Fred. *Cascade Alpine Guide*. Seattle: The Mountaineers, 1981.

Beckey, Fred. *Challenge of the North Cascades*. Seattle: The Mountaineers, 1977.

Bowers, Dan. *Exploring Garibaldi*. Vancouver: Gundy's and Bernie's Guide Books, 1972.

Bowers, Dan. *Exploring Golden Ears Park*. North Vancouver: J.J. Douglas Ltd., 1976.

Cannings, Richard and Cannings, Sydney. *British Columbia, A Natural History*. Vancouver: Greystone Books, 1996.

Cyca, Robert and Harcombe, Andrew. *Exploring Manning Park*. Vancouver: Gundy's and Bernie's Guide Books, 1973.

Decker, Frances; Fougberg, Margaret; and Ronayne, Mary. *Pemberton, The History of a Settlement*. Pemberton: Pemberton Pioneer Women, 1977.

Draycott, Walter. *Early Days in Lynn Valley*. North Vancouver: North Shore Times, 1978.

Fairley, Bruce. *A Guide to Climbing and Hiking in Southwestern British Columbia*. Vancouver: Gordon Soules, 1993.

Forsyth, Adrian. *Mammals of the Canadian Wild*. Camden East: Camdem House Publishing, 1985.

Freeman, Roger and Freeman, Ethel. *Exploring Lynn Canyon and Lynn Headwaters Park*. Vancouver: Federation of Mountain Clubs of BC, 1986.

Hull, Raymond; Soules, Gordon; and Soules, Christine. *Vancouver's Past*. Vancouver: Gordon Soules, 1974.

Jeness, Diamond. *The Faith of a Coast Salish Indian*. Victoria: BC Provincial Museum, 1955.

Johnson, Pauline. *Legends of Vancouver*. Toronto: McClelland and Stewart, 1911.

Mathews, William. *Garibaldi Geology*. Vancouver: Geological Association of Canada, 1975.

McLane, Kevin. *The Rockclimbers' Guide to Squamish*. Squamish: Merlin Productions, 1993.

McLane, Kevin. *Squamish, the Shining Valley*. Squamish: Merlin Productions, 1994.

McMahon, Anne. *The Whistler Story*. West Vancouver: A. McMahon, 1980.

Menzies, Archibald. *Menzies' Journal of Vancouver's Voyage, 1792*. Victoria: British Columbia Archives, 1923.

Morton, James. *Capilano, The Story of a River*. Toronto: McClelland and Stewart, 1970.

Munday, Don. *Mt. Garibaldi Park, Vancouver's Alpine Playground*. Vancouver: Cowan and Brookhouse, 1922.

Parish, Roberta; Coupé, Ray; and Lloyd, Dennis, eds. *Plants of Southern Interior British Columbia*. Vancouver: Lone Pine Publishing, 1996.

Peacock, Jim. *The Vancouver Natural History Society, 1918-1993*. Vancouver: Vancouver Natural History Society, 1993.

Petersen, Florence; Love Morrison, Janet; and Mitchell, Sally. *Whistler Reflections.* Vancouver: Terra Bella Publishers, 1995.

Pojar, Jim and MacKinnon, Andy, eds. *Plants of Coast British Columbia.* Vancouver: Lone Pine Publishing, 1994.

Ramsey, Bruce. *Five Corners: The Story of Chilliwack.* Chilliwack: Chilliwack Historical Society, 1975.

Stoltmann, Randy. *Hiking the Ancient Forests of British Columbia and Washington.* Vancouver: Lone Pine Publishing, 1996.

INFORMATION SOURCES

Clubs

For information on hiking clubs, contact the **Federation of Mountain Clubs of BC** at 47 West Broadway, Vancouver, BC V5Y 1P1; phone (604) 878-7007 or check the website at www.mountainclubs.bc.ca/. To learn more about the natural history of southwestern BC, check out the **Vancouver Natural History Society**, which holds regular info nights, slide shows and field trips. Contact the society at PO Box 3021, Vancouver, BC V6B 3X5, phone (604) 737-3074, website www.naaturalhistory.bc.ca/VNHS/.

Maps

Develop a love for maps. It will help keep you from getting lost and teach you much about the geography of southwestern BC. Maps range from the crude to the intricate. Collect 'em all. Here are a few places to look:

Geological Survey of Canada, 101, 605 Robson Street, Vancouver, BC V6B 5J3, phone (604) 666-0529, website www.nrcan.gc.ca/gsc. Here you'll find topographical maps of the 1:250,000, 1:50,000 scale. The bigger scale is good for an overview, the smaller more useful for navigating on the trail and for identifying specific landmarks around you.

Mountain Equipment Co-op, 130 West Broadway, Vancouver, BC V5Y 1P3; phone (604) 872–7858, website www.mec.ca. The co-op stocks some topo and other recreation maps.

International Travel Maps and Books, two stores: 530 West Broadway, Vancouver, BC V5Z 1E9, phone (604) 879-3621; 539 West Pender, Vancouver, BC V6B 1V5, phone (604) 687-3320. The website is at www.itmb.com. If you can't find the map you're looking for here, you won't find it anywhere else in town. The store has topo, recreational, urban and road maps but is a bit pricier than the above sources.

BC Parks: Maps and brochures for provincial parks are now available only online: http://wlapwww.gov.bc.ca/bcparks/index.htm. There is no general contact address, number or office for other information.

Regional Parks: For information, contact the Greater Vancouver Regional District, Parks Department at 4330 Kingsway, Burnaby, BC V5H 4G8; phone (604) 432–6350, website www.gvrd.bc.ca/services/parks/index.html.

Municipal Parks and Other Areas: For information on the hikes for **Lighthouse Park, Cypress Falls, parts of the Baden-Powell Trail** and **Brothers Creek**, contact the West Vancouver Parks Department at 750–17th Street, West Vancouver, BC V7V 3T3; phone (604) 925–7200, website www.westvancouver.net. For information on **Lynn Canyon** trails, contact the Lynn Canyon Ecology Centre at 3663 Park Road, North Vancouver, BC V7J 3G3; phone (604) 981–3103, website www.dnv.org. For information on **Stanley Park** trails, contact the Vancouver Board of Parks and Recreation at 2099 Beach Avenue, Vancouver, BC V6G 1Z4; phone (604) 257–8400, website www.city.vancouver.bc.ca/parks/.

For information on the **Buntzen Lake** and **Sendero Diez Vistas** hikes, contact BC Hydro at 6911 Southpoint Drive, Burnaby, BC V3N 4X8; phone (604) 528–1801, website www.bchydro.com/recreation/mainland/mainland1208.html.

BC Forest Service: In 2002, the government decided to phase out the BC Forest Service's recreation component, which looked after trails and campsites on land managed by the Ministry of Forests. Volunteers or a volunteer organization may eventually take over those responsibilities, and you can get information from the offices listed below.

For information on the hikes for **Blowdown Pass, Tenquille Lake, Cougar Mountain, Brandywine Meadows, Petgill Lake** and **Deeks Lake**, call the Squamish Forest District at 42000 Loggers Lane, Squamish, BC V0N 3G0, phone (604) 898-2100, website www.for.gov.bc.ca/vancouvr/district/squamish/recreation/recstart.htm.

For information on the **Mount Cheam, Vedder Ridge, Ford Mountain** and **Chilliwack River** hikes, contact the Chilliwack Forest District at 46360 Airport Road, Chilliwack, BC V2P 1A5, phone (604) 702-5700, website www.vancouvr/district/chilliwa/recreation/dck recreation.htm.

LIST OF HIKES

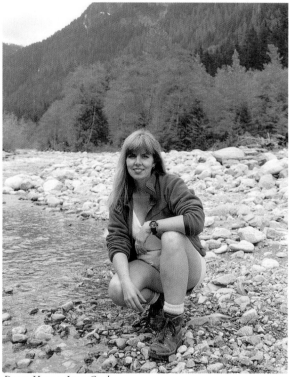
Dawn Hanna, Lynn Creek.

ABOUT THE AUTHOR

Even as a kid growing up in Kitsilano, Dawn Hanna's greatest thrills were the times spent exploring urban wilderness such as Capilano Canyon, Lighthouse Park and Mount Seymour.

Over the years, she has explored wilderness areas of BC and farther afield. She's hiked the Rockies of BC and Alberta, the Sierra Nevada mountains of California, the hills and braes of Scotland, the peaks of the Spanish Sierra Nevada, the dry interior mountains of Mexico, the rainforests and volcanoes of Hawaii and the granite and glaciers of Chile and Argentina. At-home weekends are usually spent hiking, climbing, cycling and kayaking in southern BC, sometimes with her young son Sammy. Dawn is also the author of *Easy Hikes and Walks in Southwestern BC*. She was the hiking columnist for *The Province* in Vancouver and is a freelance nature writer and media consultant.